working
with
the aged

working

MARCELLA BAKUR WEINER
Teachers College
Columbia University

ALBERT J. BROK
Postgraduate Center for Mental Health
New York, New York

ALVIN M. SNADOWSKY
Brooklyn College
of the City University of New York

with the aged

practical
approaches
in
the institution
and community

Prentice-Hall, Inc., Englewood Cliffs, N.J. 07632

Library of Congress Cataloging in Publication Data

Weiner, Marcella B (date)
   Working with the aged.

   Includes bibliographical references and index.
   1. Geriatric nursing.   2. Aged—Rehabilitation.
I. Brok, Albert J., joint author.   II. Snadowsky,
Alvin M., (date) joint author.   III. Title.
RC954.W39   610.73'65   77-29154
ISBN 0-13-967570-1

working with the aged:
practical approaches in the institution and community
Marcella Bakur Weiner, Albert J. Brok, and Alvin M. Snadowsky

1139479

HV 1461
W

Printed in the United States of America

10 9 8 7 6 5 4 3 2 1

PRENTICE-HALL INTERNATIONAL, INC., *London*
PRENTICE-HALL OF AUSTRALIA PTY. LIMITED, *Sydney*
PRENTICE-HALL OF CANADA, LTD., *Toronto*
PRENTICE-HALL OF INDIA PRIVATE LIMITED, *New Delhi*
PRENTICE-HALL OF JAPAN, INC., *Tokyo*
PRENTICE-HALL OF SOUTHEAST ASIA PTE. LTD., *Singapore*
WHITEHALL BOOKS LIMITED, *Wellington, New Zealand*

contents

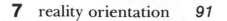

preface

The primary purpose of this book is to provide guidelines, techniques, and approaches for working with older people in institutional and community settings. This book was written because we believe that the physical and psychosocial characteristics of older people are unique enough to merit approaches tailored to their needs. We hope that this book will stimulate new ways of thinking about working with people who are experiencing both the virtues and difficulties inherent in the later stages of life.

This book contains a theoretical base and a practical approach geared to helping the older person. The more practical aspects offer step-by-step guides for setting up and implementing various rehabilitation and group-counseling techniques. Thus, the novice, as well as the experienced worker, is given a clear understanding of implementing such tasks as which patient to select; how to arrange a room suited for a particular technique; and how to deal with problems which may arise.

Since the techniques described are still relatively new, we cannot provide definitive, empirical proof that they work. However, our clinical experience, as well as that of the many students and colleagues with whom we have worked, suggests that the methods described are very effective. It is our hope that people entering or working in the field of aging will try these techniques, and in doing so, modify and improve them, as we ourselves do continually. Further, it is our desire that some of our more provocative ideas will stimulate research programs to validate systematically the clinical basis of our methods.

Throughout this book, the word *he* has been used in the

generic sense to include both men and women.

Our appreciation is extended to all the elderly with whom we worked whose needs prompted this book; to our professional colleagues whose constructive advice spurred us on; and to our family members whose support and enthusiasm were so invaluable.

We are indebted to Matthew Gold, Patricia Nolan, and Winifred Warner, Rehabilitation Specialists, for their guidance and contributions to the sections on the institutionalized aged; and to Miriam Aronson of Columbia University who reviewed portions of the manuscript and made contributions from her many years of experience in working with older people. Gratitude is also extended to Dorie Greenspan of Columbia University and Delores Herzog who provided research assistance and inspiration. We are particularly indebted to William Gibson of Prentice-Hall for his support and editorial guidance. We thank William Weiner and Carol Brok, mental health practitioners, for invaluable professional and personal support.

A special debt of gratitude is owed to staff personnel at the David Minkin Rehabilitation Institute, who, under the administration of Mr. Harris Brodsky, implemented the institutional techniques described.

Finally, our deep thanks to Rita Roth whose skillful typing of our manuscript made life much simpler for all of us.

Marcella Bakur Weiner
Albert J. Brok
Alvin M. Snadowsky

I

an
overview

1

why work
with
the aged?

Looking at One's Own Aging

Most young people do not think about old age. Rather, it is pushed
into the back of the mind where it becomes one of the "some day,
when I . . ." stems to be completed at a much later date. Yet, the
feelings we have about our own aging process and our own old age
play a large part in determining whether or not we want to work
with older people. Most importantly, this attitude has a direct
bearing on how effectively we work with the older person. Persons
in the field of aging usually agree that it is this interaction between
the patient and worker that is most related to beneficial change in
the patient, i.e., to any potential "cure." Those of us who have a
positive, accepting view of our own aging are more able to offer
compassion, empathy, concern, and appropriate support to our
patients; the others communicate to their patients their own
anxieties, fears, and overconcerns of aging no matter how well they
attempt to mask their feelings. Fearing one's own aging and
working face to face each day with aging persons would also seem a
less than optimal working condition!

Most young students entering the "helping professions" do
not choose to work with the older person. Wilensky and Barmack
designed a behavior preference questionnaire to assess the
attitudes of clinical psychology doctoral students toward working
with the aging. Responses were received from psychology doctoral
students in six universities in the New York City area. The authors
report strikingly similar response patterns for all six universities,
with greatest preference directed toward working with young

adults and a tendency for respondents to avoid working with the elderly.[1]

In our youth-oriented society all that is new, novel, and fresh is to be desired; being old is equated with loss, illness, and eventual death. Why then work with the old? What benefits can be gained by the patient and by the worker?

Old People Can Change

In order to gain satisfaction from working with people, the worker needs to feel that he has had an impact on the person seeking help. This positive change in the patient helps confirm and reinforce the worker's own sense of effectiveness. Although much of society's projected image of the old person is that he is incapable of change or that "it is all organic," those working with the aged, in whatever setting, dispute this. Thus, the authors, for example, have seen patients, in their 80's and 90's being discharged from an institution as a result of positive changes in their physical and psychological status attributed, in part, as a consequence of therapeutic efforts. This may be replicated by noticeable positive changes in patients, also in their later years, who have come for psychological counseling or psychotherapy. Thus, old people, like young and middle-aged people, can be helped to change if *both* they and the worker believe that this help is possible. This belief may be the most essential link toward promoting change.

Quality versus Quantity

Though the older person is closer to the end of his life than the younger one, the worker must feel that helping a person live out the rest of his years more satisfactorily, even if those years are limited in number, is a most worthwhile endeavor. The quality of a life's experience cannot be measured in the same way as quantity, but numbers of years may have little to do with satisfactions in living. The only possible way to help measure relieving another person's human suffering and/or to help make life better for him would be in terms of one's own internalized value system, i.e., a

---

[1]H. Wilensky and J. Barmack, "Interests of Doctoral Students in Clinical Psychology in Work with Older Adults," *Journal of Gerontology* **21** (1966): 410–414.

sense of one's own feelings of accomplishment and heightened self-esteem through reaching out and offering assistance to another. The quality of this experience, regardless of its time span, will then be felt and appreciated not only by the patient but also by the worker himself. Only this form of mutuality leads to positive change in both.

Old People Appreciate Help

The older population is often a population in need. Experiencing physical and psychosocial declines, the older person is often in need of some kind of help. This dependency often reflects itself in the depth and intensity of the appreciation extended to the worker, the one who is "there for me." When offered assistance, the patient's first comment may be "Why bother with me when there are younger people around to help?" No doubt, this is a reflection on society's values that attention is focused on the young. If, however, one can go beyond this overt verbalization and initial resistance and sincerely reach out to help, gratitude is huge. This gratitude acts as a positive reinforcer that deepens one's own sense of self-worth and professional and personal competence. Being thanked by the patient confirms that one is wanted and needed. In addition, the experience of change in the patient reconfirms the worker's belief that life at any stage involves continued growth and development.

Practical Considerations

It is common knowledge that all Americans are living longer, i.e., that longevity is on the increase. Therefore, the need for persons in the field of aging is also on the rise. Thus, the field of aging still offers work opportunities. One has only to look in the employment section of any newspaper to note this. Thus, "arming" oneself with skills and insights for working with this age group would appear to be consistent with needed services and societal trends. The aged are here to stay and they are here to stay longer. We should be prepared to work with them.

Your Own Qualities and Growth Experience

There are still relatively little data on qualities needed to make one effective in working with the older person. In a study by Conte,

Weiner, Plutchik, Bennett, and White seeking to discriminate between nurses' aides who were considered by their supervisors to be successful or unsuccessful in working with older patients, the authors found that successful aides ranked higher on qualities of patience, acceptance, flexibility, tolerance, and respect.[2] Certain factors may appear self-evident, such as that the older person is usually slower in his responses and, therefore, requires more time to complete a task. Similarly, not accepted as a full citizen by a society that is geared to the young, he would do best with a worker/therapist who shows a good degree of acceptance and respect for his many years of living. In addition, were the worker to have a flexibility of style, this could act as a modifier toward what may be perceived as the older person's "rigidity" but which, upon closer examination, is often a need for preserving and clinging tightly to that which is familiar.

How then does one evaluate the extent of these qualities in one's self? The answer may be only by trying to get in touch with the feelings one has toward working with the older adult, by reflecting upon, examining, and accepting these feelings, of whatever nature. The adage of "being true to yourself" could not be more apt!

If one does conclude that he is motivated to work with the aging person, he will find that the satisfactions are many. Primary to this are satisfactions related to the worker's own growth experience. Those in the field of psychotherapy, in particular, have written much on the interaction between the patient and the therapist. Stress is placed on the fact that much of the patient's improvement is contingent on his relationship with "a new object," i.e., the therapist.[3] In addition, change can also come about in the worker/therapist if he is in tune with not only the patient's world but his own, the therapist's, as well. Thus, by his interactions with his patient, the worker can become a more integrated, better functioning, better feeling person. This may partially come about through empathic understanding and mutual identifications. That is, the older patient may see in the younger worker both his own youthful past and possibilities for the future; the worker, often younger, may see in the patient portions of his own aging. In this way, each may be able to foresee and possibly play out a trial fantasy

---

[2]H. Conte, M. B. Weiner, R. Plutchik, R. Bennett, and M. White, "Selecting Successful Workers with Aged Persons: An Empirical Investigation," paper presented at the 46th annual meeting of the Eastern Psychological Association, New York, 1975.

[3]H. W. Loewald, "On the Therapeutic Action of Psycho-analysis," *International Journal of Psychoanalysis* **41** (1960): 16–33.

for a phase of one's own future existence. This integration of past and present with the future provides both patient and worker with a most viable frame of reference for living. It may serve as the base for optimal growth experiences.

2

physiological aging

Although we all begin the aging process at conception, the point in time at which we classify ourselves or find ourselves classified by society as "being old" can vary tremendously. Who the aged are and how and when they are identified as such depend on and involve an understanding of the various ways the aging process is conceptualized. Thus, aging may be narrowly viewed in terms of particular physical characteristics and biological processes or it may be more broadly viewed from social, cultural, legal, psychological, or experiential perspectives. More often than not, all of the above perspectives, whether broad or narrow, have a place in defining the category "aged." Indeed, it is only through understanding the interrelationships among the various perspectives that we can truly comprehend what is meant by the concept "growing old." In this and in the following chapter we shall discuss some of the ways of defining *who are the aged* and consider issues relevant to each definition as well as to their integration.

What are the signs of aging? What is normal aging? Are there basic physiological processes that change with age in the absence of disease? What limits the length of human life? These are some of the critical issues involved in defining *who the aged are* in biological terms.

Signs of Aging

Perhaps the most apparent signs of aging involve the appearance of changes in a person's physical characteristics. Thus, the gradual emergence of graying hair and skin wrinkles, the loss of teeth, poor eyesight, decreased hearing acuity, and various postural changes are all signs that seem to give clear and unequivocal indications of a person's age. However, we must also point out that such changes are not directly correlated with any specific *chronological age* but are subject to wide individual differences.[1]

To many, chronological age (our actual age in years) is the principal sign of old age. Thus, it is common in the American culture to consider anyone who has reached the age of 65 as "old." Although chronological age is a good general indicator of physical abilities, it leaves a lot to be desired as a basis for making assumptions about any particular individual's physical health or any particular person's sense of psychological well-being. The person who "looks old" may not "feel old" or, for that matter, even be old in chronological terms. On the other hand, an individual whose physical appearance indicates a "youthful" 65 may feel very depressed about his chronological age.

There is little doubt that the relationship between general functioning and chronological age is strongly modified by individual differences. Although there is an abundance of research showing that the most characteristic sign of advanced chronological age is a decline in the speed of both mental and physical functioning, a number of exceptions to this generalization have been observed. Jarvik, for example, repeatedly tested one older female during a 20-year period (from age 60 to 80) and reported no decline in scores on a tapping test;[2] whereas research with elderly drivers showed that many of them had reaction times comparable to young drivers, although on the *average* they were slower than the younger drivers.[3] Similarly, Botwinick and Thompson observed no differences in reaction time between 68- to 86-year-old males and a group of males 18 to 22 years when the younger group were not particularly athletic. These researchers suggest that such extrinsic factors as amount of daily exercise, rather than decrements associated with chronological age, could in part account for observed similarities or differences between age groups in reaction times.[4] In fact, it has been noted that the extent of individual differences is so great that many older subjects can be

[1]L. F. Jarvik, "Thoughts on the Psychobiology of Aging," *American Psychologist* **30** (1975): 576–583.

[2]Ibid.

[3]D. T. Giantucco, D. Ramm, and C. W. Erwin, "The Elderly Driver and Ex-driver," in *Normal Aging II,* ed., E. Palmore (Durham, N.C.: Duke University Press, 1974): 173–179.

[4]J. Botwinick and L. W. Thompson, "Cardiac Functioning and Reaction Time in Relation to Age," *Journal of Genetic Psychology* **119** (1971): 127–132.

observed to perform more quickly than younger subjects in laboratory reaction time experiments.[5]

Normal Aging and Disease States

One difficulty in describing the process of *normal aging* from a biological perspective is that many of the physical and biological changes observed with increasing age may be the results of disease states related to age rather than to the aging process itself. Although research shows that human cells grown in laboratory cultures seem to have a limited capacity to duplicate,[6] and that individuals experience a decline in integrated body functions at the rate of approximately 1 percent a year, many scientists continue to believe that no one really dies of "old age." Rather, death is caused by specific diseases or disorders that are in some way correlated with old age, i.e., aging may be a process that increases the probability of disease.[7]

The problem of clearly distinguishing between "abnormal" disorders that can be treated medically and/or psychologically and changes that are inevitable as a result of age is a long-standing one. For example, if we look at assumptions of old age throughout history, we can see that the process of normal aging has often been confused with the process of disease and decline. Since many of the program designs and activities suggested for working with or rehabilitating the aged are based on assumptions about *what* might be expected from the "normal aged," it becomes extremely important to distinguish between the biases handed down from history and factual material about the aging process. In this framework, let us now look at some of the theories of normal aging offered throughout the past. We shall also discuss how these theories might have an effect on current program ideals and goals.

Theories of Normal Aging in the Past

Since ancient times the concept of aging as an inevitable and normal process of decline, similar to that of a disease state, has been

---

[5]J. Botwinick, *Aging and Behavior* (New York: Springer, 1973).

[6]L. Hayflick, "Aging under Glass," *Experimental Gerontology* 5 (1970): 291–304.

[7]E. L. Bierman and W. R. Hazzard, "Biology of Aging," in *The Biologic Ages of Man, from Conception through Old Age,* eds., D. W. Smith and E. L. Bierman (Philadelphia: W. B. Saunders Co., 1973).

considered the most basic explanation for growing old. Perhaps
this is because of the historical connection between the emergence
of medical science and the study of aging.[8] For example, one of the
earliest biologically oriented theories of aging was generated by
Hippocrates, the Greek philosopher and the father of modern
medicine. He believed that old age was caused by the progressive
imbalance in what was then thought of as the four basic body
substances—blood, phlegm, choler, and black choler.
Interestingly, these imbalances were also thought to be the cause of
sickness. Thus, it seems clear that Hippocrates tended to view the
process of aging as caused by the same factors as illness. The Greek
philosopher–scientist was also the first to express the stages of
human development in terms of the four seasons, with old age, as
we might expect, relegated to winter.[9] The winter analogy remains
a popular symbol today and underlies the biologically oriented
conception of the inevitability of aging as being equal to decline.
During the middle ages, old age was also generally looked upon as
an incurable disease, and even during the Renaissance the growth
of interest in human anatomy and science in general did not seem
to greatly change basic conceptions of the aging process.[10]

   Since the Renaissance many physical and biological oriented
theories of aging have been generated. Perhaps two of the most
significant of these can be termed the *wear and tear theory* and the
declining energy theory. As all theories, these two tend to be based on
the prevailing philosophical conception of man at a particular
point in the historical development of a culture. In terms of the
aging process, this means that *how* aging is understood is in part
dependent on *what* we believe is responsible for human
functioning. By studying some of these prevailing philosophical
conceptions, we can perhaps gain an understanding of the
rationale behind various programs, goals, and ideals developed for
working with the aged. In this light, we turn to brief descriptions of
the wear and tear and declining energy theories.

wear and tear theory: man as a machine

   Although the viewpoint that man is essentially similar to a
complex mechanical device whose parts are replaceable can be

---

[8]S. de Beauvoir, *The Coming of Age* (New York: G. P. Putnam's Sons, 1972).
[9]Ibid.
[10]Ibid.

traced back to classical times—such as when Aristotle noted that an old man needed only the eye of a young man in order to look like a young man[11]—the concept of *man as a machine* has continued to be important throughout history. This concept especially seems to have gained popularity during the eighteenth and nineteenth centuries with the emergence of the philosophical school of rationalism. Descartes, for example, in believing that the mind and body were separate, argued that the body functions operated essentially as a complex machine.[12] In the field of medicine this sort of thinking had great influence on a group of scientists called *iatrophysicists.*

Iatrophysics was a school of medicine especially popular in the eighteenth century that attempted to combine the concepts of mechanical physics with medicine. Specifically, scientists of this school tried to explain both disease processes and activities of the body in terms of physics instead of chemistry. To the iatrophysicists, the process of normal aging occurred as a result of body deterioration—just as a machine wears out when it has been used too long.[13]

This wear and tear theory remains popular today. We only have to think of the hope that many people have about the possibility that organ transplants can insure longevity by means of replacing "the old used up parts of the body" with new functional ones in order to note the continuing impact of the wear and tear theory. Unfortunately, the "spare parts" concept inherent in such a theory does not seem to be plausible as a method for increasing the life span. It appears that specific organ transplants do not seem to affect the apparent decline with age in the efficiency of complex homeostatic mechanisms, or the process of cellular aging.[14]

Implications of the wear and tear theory. From a social point of view, we believe that the continuing impact of the wear and tear theory can still be observed as a subtle influence on the program goals and the ideals of those working with the aged. Machines are things of motion. They function best when kept running at a steady pace. Inactivity or disuse can lead to rust and

---

[11]G. A. Zilboorg, *A History of Medical Psychology* (New York: W. W. Norton and Company, 1941).

[12]W. Kohler, *The Task of Gestalt Psychology* (Princeton, N.J.: Princeton University Press, 1969).

[13]S. de Beauvoir, *The Coming of Age.*

[14]D. C. Kimmel, *Adulthood and Aging* (New York: John Wiley and Sons, 1974).

need for replacement. When such thinking is translated into life-style values it is very reflective of the prevailing ~~American~~ ethic of "keep active, keep busy, keep in motion."

Thus, it was perhaps no accidental finding when a recent sociological survey revealed a 73-year-old man as saying that his main goal in life is to "keep active—I want to wear out, not rust out."[15] This fear of "rusting," of the machine wearing down, may be a major psychological issue for many older Americans. The overidentification with machine-type attributes may in turn lead to an overemphasis on compulsive activity or "doing" patterns and, in turn, to a de-emphasis on the value of contemplation, leisure, or "being" states. Social scientists, for example, have indicated that Americans do not as a rule take easily (or readily) to leisure when it is made available in the form of retirement.[16]

In light of the above, we might also note that critiques by Eastern (e.g., Indian) psychiatric viewpoints of American and Western style therapies include the notion that Americans tend not to enjoy the simple experience of "being" with each other but feel that they must "get or achieve something" out of doing things with each other.[17] Such notions, buried deep in the American ethic of the need for achievement, when combined with an identification with mechanistic analogies of man often form the basis for program goals and ideals that roughly follow the dictates of the *activity theory*.

Basically, this theory involves the notion that "if you keep busy, you stay healthy." As we shall subsequently note in the section on the Community Aged, such thinking may lead to activity programs in which thoughts about *what* old people keep busy *with* may be less important than the *mere activity* of keeping busy. When uncritically accepted (although certainly of some benefit), the attitude that people should be kept "busy" can lead workers and programmers to erroneously overfocus on the *number* of activities while diminishing concern for the *quality* of the activities. It also can lead to a diminished concern with the quality of the relationship experiences engendered by a program in deference to a "numbers count" attitude. Quantity of social acquaintances does not necessarily mean good quality of friendship experiences.

---

[15]V. L. Bengston, *The Social Psychology of Aging* (New York: Bobbs-Merrill, 1973), p. 6.

[16]R. J. Havighurst, "Social Roles, Work, Leisure, and Education," in *The Psychology of Adult Development and Aging,* eds., C. Eisdorfer and M. O. Lawton (Washington, D.C.: American Psychological Association, 1973).

[17]S. K. Pande, "The Mystique of 'Western' Psychotherapy: An Eastern Interpretation," *The Journal of Nervous and Mental Disease* **146** (1968): 425–432.

declining energy theory:
man as having limited vitality

The concept of man as a biological energy system, as if he were a dry cell battery that could not be recharged, is implicit in various theories of aging. For example, aging has been conceptualized as involving a progressive decline of vigor and resistance with the passage of time[18] or as a decline in physiological competence that both increases and intensifies the effects of various forms of environmental stress.[19] Two important notions about the aging process emerge from the following definitions:

1. Aging implies a decline in either energy or vigor.
2. This decline in vigor results in a lower ability to deal with outside forces (lessened resistance and tolerance of environmental stress).

The idea that aging implies some sort of innate or other energy decline is partially derived from the philosophy of *vitalism*. The vitalists were early biologists and philosophers who were not content with the purely physical theories of life popular during the middle ages. In particular, they believed that life was at least in some part self-determining instead of mechanistically determined, and they, therefore, postulated the existence of an energy source that was nonphysical. The existence of this nonphysical energy source, or *vital principle*, was thought to "use" the physical apparatus of the body, such as the nerves, muscles, and specialized organs, as a means to act on the natural world.[20] The vitalistic assumption indicates that the gradual loss of this energy over time, and its ultimate disappearance, is what brings about old age and eventually death.[21] It is interesting to note that a similar notion was implicit in Freud's theory of libido—an instinctual energy that conceivably dissipates with age.[22]

Variations on the idea of declining energy as an explanation

---

[18]Bierman and Hazzard, "Biology of Aging."

[19]P. S. Timiras, *Developmental Physiology and Aging* (New York: Macmillan Publishing Company, 1972).

[20]S. K. Langer, *Mind: An Essay on Human Feeling* (Baltimore, Md.: The John Hopkins Press, 1967).

[21]S. de Beauvoir, *The Coming of Age.*

[22]S. Freud, *An Outline of Psycho-Analysis* (New York: W. W. Norton and Company, 1969).

for the process of aging have not been confined to Western
European thinking. For example, Holmberg noted that various
Andean tribal groups have the following belief on aging:

> ... the human organism has in its constitution a given number of
> ounces of earth. The quantity, although fixed for the individual,
> varies from person to person. Some have more; others less. The
> existence of strong and weak people, in fact, is explained on the basis
> that some people have more earth in their constitutions than others.
> Those having the greatest amount are also those who show the
> greatest physical resistance on such occasions as drinking feasts and
> religious festivals which are popular and widespread institutions in
> the Andes.[23]

Thus, although never proved, assumptions about aging
related to or derived from vitalistic notions have maintained their
appeal over many centuries. In modern times they exemplify the
battery analogy of man, i.e., that we have a fixed amount of energy
that we use up (or run out of) over time.

Implications of the declining energy theory.   The belief
that people have a limited amount of vitality that dissipates with age
may still continue to exert influences on both theories of aging and
practices of working with the aged. For example, those working
with the aged might tend to believe that old people prefer to
disengage from society, i.e., that they prefer to be left alone, to
reminisce or introspect about the past instead of engaging in
face-to-face interaction in the environment. Cumming and Henry,
for example, have proposed a formalized *disengagement theory of
aging* based on data obtained from a sample of Kansas City
elderly.[24] In their sample they found that chronological aging was
accompanied by a steady decline in social interaction, ego, and
energy involvement in the social environment and by a decline in
role activity. From these and related data it has been proposed that
normal successful aging involves a mutual disengagement
between the individual and society. The disengagement theory
implies that the sources of psychological well-being in old age are
substantially different from those of middle age, which are
assumed to be more dependent on high levels of social activity and

---

[23]A. R. Holmberg, "Age in the Andes," in *Aging and Leisure*, ed. R. W. Kleemeir (New York: Oxford University Press, 1961), pp. 86–87.

[24]E. Cumming and W. E. Henry, *Growing Old: The Process of Disengagement* (New York: Basic Books, 1961).

social–interpersonal interaction.[25] In sum, the disengagement theory encourages those who work with the aged to believe that much interest and involvement in the "outer world" should not be expected from old people. This sort of thinking can subtly influence policy and program goals to de-emphasize remotivational-type programs that encourage continued exploration and interest in the environment. Such thinking may also serve as a rationalization to maintain forced retirement policies and to discourage retraining those who are already retired.

Further research on the disengagement theory seems to indicate that the process of normal psychologically successful aging is not solely related to the need for a timely mutual disengagement of the individual and the society. Instead, it is strongly determined and moderated by individual personality characteristics.[26] In sum, Neugarten, Havighurst, and Tobin note:

> People, as they grow old, seem to be neither at the mercy of the social environment nor at the mercy of some set of intrinsic processes—in either instance, inexorable changes that they cannot influence. On the contrary, the individual seems to continue to make his own "impress" upon the wide range of social and biological changes. He continues to exercise choice and to select from the environment in accordance with his own long-established needs. He ages according to a pattern that has a long history, and that maintains itself, with adaptation, to the end of life.[27]

We believe that it is important for those who work or create programs for the aged to be sensitive to the individual characteristics of the elderly as suggested above.

Distinguishing Between Normal Aging and Disease States in Recent Times

As we have seen, the problem of clearly distinguishing between abnormal disorders that are to be treated and changes that are "inevitable" as a result of age has been a long-standing one throughout history. The ability to draw such clear-cut distinctions still remains a difficult task.

---

[25]Bengston, *The Social Psychology of Aging.*

[26]B. L. Neugarten, R. J. Havighurst, and S. S. Tobin, "Personality and Patterns of Aging," in *Middle Age and Aging*, eds., B. L. Neugarten (Chicago: The University of Chicago Press, 1968).

[27]Ibid., p. 177.

The problem of correctly assessing age differences in blood pressure is one simple example of the current difficulty in discriminating between disease states and the normal aging process. As we grow older, measurements of diastolic and particularly systolic blood pressure tend to be higher than when we were younger. Hypertension, which is associated with high blood pressure, is also a physical sign of a number of serious diseases that can be medically treated. When faced with these facts, health professionals have to decide whether observed high blood pressure in an older individual should be medically treated or considered normal. Underlying such a decision is the problem of deciding on whether standards of normality for blood pressure should be adjusted for age.[28] On this and related issues Bierman and Hazzard note:

> Blood pressure is only one of many examples of the principle that the change in organ function with age may be indistinguishable in magnitude, direction, and character from the change in function which occurs in well-defined disease states. Tests of pulmonary or renal function clearly demonstrate progressive decrements with increasing age which resemble the common chronic pulmonary and renal diseases. In these instances, however, where therapy [medical treatment] is by *no* means as effective or as readily evaluated as in the hypertensive diseases and where the measurements themselves are not as simple to perform, the relation of age change to disease has *not* become as pressing a problem. [However, let us] . . . consider also the condition of prostatism. Here our ability to quantitate the change with age [or disease?] is *poor* indeed and the therapy, surgery, not one to be undertaken lightly. . . . The point to be made by these examples is that the conditions of a particular historical moment strongly influence the physician's view toward aging and disease.[29]

Thus we can see that even today it is not a simple matter to clearly distinguish the aging process from the process of disease.

Some Basic Physiological Processes that Change with Age in the Absence of Disease

homeostasis

Although we may not be able to specify the exact cause of aging, we can describe various changes that seem to occur along

---

[28]E. L. Bierman and W. R. Hazzard, "Old Age, Including Death and Dying," in *The Biologic Ages of Man, from Conception through Old Age,* eds., Smith and Bierman.
[29]Ibid., pp. 174–175.

with age. For example, the body's ability to regulate levels of blood
ph, blood sugar, and pulse rate under various and changing
conditions seems to decline with age. In general, research shows
that there is almost a linear decline of approximately 1 percent a
year in most integrated body functions in adult life.[30] Despite these
facts, it also has been shown that old people maintain basic
homeostatic balances (the way the body stabilized its physiological
functioning) as efficiently as younger persons under resting
conditions. What seems to be problematical is that advanced age
greatly impairs the body's capacity to favorably readjust internal
functioning after experiencing stressful circumstances.[31] This
decline in the body's ability to maintain a proper homeostatic
balance in the face of stress may be considered one of the major
problems of normal aging. Some scientists, for example, have
estimated that if we kept the same resistance and resilience to stress
throughout our life span that we had at age 12, then half of us alive
today could expect to live another 700 years.[32]

The likelihood that old people react more severely to stress
than younger people carries implications for programming and
working with the aged. Thus, techniques used in working with the
aged should perhaps minimize or take into account the "excitatory
potential" or stress of the social and physical environment. For
example, we have elsewhere outlined the various problem source
areas and stresses to which old people are especially vulnerable.
Briefly summarized, these involve decreases in sensory capacities
and physical mobility, the loss of status and shrinkage of roles,
various psychological life crises engendered by realization of the
loss of youth, and philosophical crises induced by thoughts about
the general meaning of life. Thus, the stresses to which the aged
are susceptible can come from many sources. "Best fit" models of
treatment should take into account the source of each particular
stress as well as how the individual aged person copes with each
stress.

cell loss

Until recently the theory that aging involves the progressive
loss of cells was widely accepted. Cell loss was thought to be
responsible for decreased muscular strength, impairment of brain
functioning, and other symptoms of old age. The greatest loss of

---

[30]Ibid.

[31]Kimmel, *Adulthood and Aging.*

[32]Bierman and Hazzard, "Biology of Aging."

cells in humans seems to occur in the brain, skeletal muscles, and kidneys, with some loss found in the liver.[33] Although still of some importance, cell loss is not currently considered a crucial factor in normal aging.

cell and tissue aging

In opposition to the decreasing importance of cell loss as a factor in aging there is a strong controversy about the effects of cellular aging. One of the basic issues here is whether or not human cells have a finite life span. One fascinating group of findings reported by Hayflick seems to indicate that cells *do* have a definite life span. He reports that cells grown in laboratory cultures die out after 50 doublings.[34] Bierman and Hazzard also indicate that human cells grown in tissue culture do not divide indefinitely but instead show a decreasing capacity for finite division with age. They note that cells taken from a human embryo divide about 50 times in culture while those taken from a 20-year-old duplicate about 30 times. In comparison, cells obtained from older donors divide about 20 times.[35] The propensity for cells to be limited by some finite duplication appears to occur across animal species. For example, comparison of aging of normal cells derived from different animal species also shows that considerable differences exist between species, with man being second to the Galapagos tortoise. Table 2.1 summarizes the available data on cross-species differences.

Does all this mean that the mechanism for aging is to be found in the finiteness of cell duplication? Unfortunately, the answer is not clear because we do not know if cells in a laboratory culture act the same way that cells in a living functioning organism would. Another aspect of the controversy lies within the research itself. Kohn reports on a number of studies that conflict with the model and results proposed by Hayflick. These studies seem to indicate that there is "no clear generalized age-associated loss of cell ability to divide (in mammals) followed by the dying out of these cells."[36]

---

[33]L. F. Jarvik and D. Cohen, "A Biobehavioral Approach to Intellectual Changes with Aging," in *The Psychology of Adult Development and Aging,* eds., Eisdorfer and Lawton.

[34]L. Hayflick, "Why Grow Old?" *The Stanford Magazine* **3** (1975): 36–43.

[35]Bierman and Hazzard, "Biology of Aging."

[36]R. R. Kohn, "Aging and Cell Division," *Science* **188** (1975): 204.

Table 2.1 The finite lifetime of cultured normal embryonic human and animal fibroblasts*

Species	Range of Population Doublings for Cultured Normal Embryo Fibroblasts (Cells)	Mean Maximum Life Span in Years
Galapagos tortoise	90–125	175 (?)
Man	40–60	110
Mink	30–34	10
Chicken	15–35	30 (?)
Mouse	14–28	3.5

Adapted from L. Hayflick, "Why Grow Old?" *The Stanford Magazine* **3** (1975): 36–43.

aging at the molecular level

There are some who believe that the aging process may be the result of the accumulation of "errors" in "the genetic matrix which generates the many physiochemical systems supporting cell biosynthesis and homeostatic regulation."[37] Specifically, it seems that problems arise over time in the genetically programmed DNA–RNA enzyme protein synthesis necessary for the proper functioning of cells. [DNA (deoxyribonucleic acid) determines the formation of RNA (ribonucleic acid) which, in turn, produces enzymes involved in cellular functioning.] The errors that might occur include mutations, cross-linkages, incorrect transcription (the formation of RNA from DNA), etc. All of these factors can create *creeping error* in the cell system and contribute to the production of *anamolus* protein.[38] Such cumulative errors may be a major source of changes leading to senescence.[39]

Unfortunately, scientists disagree on why the changes alluded to above occur. There are those who argue that these changes are evolutionary in nature while others believe that these problems

[37] Jarvik and Cohen, "A Biobehavioral Approach to Intellectual Changes with Aging," p. 234.

[38] Ibid.

[39] L. E. Orgel, "The Maintenance of the Accuracy of Protein Synthesis and Its Relevance to Aging," *Proceedings of the National Academy of Sciences* **49** (1963): 517–521.

"are essentially random events that accumulate with age until the cell itself becomes defective."[40]

autoimmunity and accumulation
of metabolic waste

Various other theories on the aging process have been proposed. One involves the notion that aging occurs because cells are slowly poisoned by metabolic waste products that accumulate over time. Another theory proposes that over time the body builds up immunity to its own tissues through the production of autoimmune antibodies. This process would theoretically lead to cell dysfunction and death. However, these theories are generally unproven and are considered to be symptoms rather than causes of aging.[41]

---

[40]Kimmel, *Adulthood and Aging*, p. 355.
[41]Ibid.

psychological aging

Aspects of Normal Personality Development in Old Age

Although it has been generally acknowledged throughout history that people continue to develop and change as they grow older, there were relatively little psychological data on the latter half of the life cycle that was systematically organized prior to the early part of the twentieth century. Until the 1920's the comprehension of personality in later life had not moved much beyond Shakespeare's classic statement on the seven ages of man.

> All the world's a stage,
> And all the men and women merely players;
> They have their exits and their entrances,
> And one man in his time plays many parts,
> His acts being seven ages. At first the infant . . .
> Then the whining schoolboy . . .
> Creeping like a snail,
>   Unwillingly to school. And then the lover,
> Sighing like a furnace . . .
> Then a soldier,
> Full of strange oaths and bearded like the pard,
> Jealous in honor, sudden and quick in quarrel,
> Seeking the bubble reputation,
> Even in the cannon's mouth. And then the justice . . .
> With eyes severe and beard of formal cut,
> Full of wise saws and modern instances . . .
>   The sixth age shifts

Into the lean and slippered pantaloon,
With spectacles on nose and pouch on side;
His youthful hose, well saved, a world too wide
For his shrunk shank, and his big manly voice,
Turning again toward childish treble, pipes
And whistles in his sound. Last scene of all,
That ends this strange eventful history,
Is second childishness and mere oblivion,
Sans teeth, sans eyes, sans taste, sans everything.

As You Like It

Shakespeare's belief that old age was equivalent to an empty "second childishness and mere oblivion" may still be considered true by some of those working with the aged because of the nature of some of the simple activity programs made available to many of our senior citizens. Fortunately, there seems to be more to old age than Shakespeare would have us believe. In this light, we shall now briefly consider some of the prominent theories and concepts that relate to personality development in later life.

Bühler: self-fulfillment
and life goals in later life

The Viennese psychologist Charlotte Bühler was one of the first researchers to actually gather data on issues faced in old age. She collected life histories in autobiographical form from elderly people.[1] In the present context, Bühler's principal contribution was the suggestion that the life span can be divided into various phases or stages that do not completely parallel (but rather are similar to) the biological life course of growth, stability, and decline. Implicit in her findings were the notions that mental abilities such as intelligence do not decline as rapidly as physical capacities and that old age may be a time for continued goal development and concerns about self-fulfillment. Interviews with old people showed that fulfillment in old age often involved the following four major considerations:

   1. *The aspect of luck:* Fufilled people almost always seem to mention that their life involved meeting the right persons, or

---

[1] C. Bühler, *Der Menschliche Lebenslauf als Psychologisches Problem* (Leipzig: Herzel, 1933; 2nd ed., Gottingen: Verlag fuer Psychologie, 1959); C. Bühler, "The Curve of Life as Studies in Biographies," *Journal of Applied Psychology* 19 (1953): 405–409; C. Bühler, "Human Life Goals in the Humanistic Perspective," *Journal of Humanistic Psychology* 7 (1967): 36–52.

being at the right place at the right time. Religious persons view this as the work of God. Unfufilled people view their life as marked by bad luck.

2. *Feelings about the realization of one's potentialities:* Fufilled people note that "I did most of what I wanted to do," or "I did what was right for me." Unfufilled people display the opposite feelings.

3. *The aspect of accomplishment:* The feeling that "there was something to show" for one's past life is a major contributing factor to feelings of satisfaction or dissatisfaction in later life.

4. *Moral evaluation:* Individuals who seem fulfilled tend to emphasize that they "had lived right"—this is meant in terms of their religious or moral convictions. Fulfilled people seem to emphasize that they had dedicated themselves to some highly valued objective in family relations or had made progress in some important field of endeavor, or given their support to various social groups.[2]

In general, Bühler's personality-oriented suggestions about the achievement of fulfillment in later life were believed by her to be more critical for psychological adjustment in old age than either biological decline or the experiences of insecurity engendered by social losses.

Jung: the process of individuation in later life

C. G. Jung was one of the first psychiatrists to break from total agreement with Freudian theory. The emphasis Freud placed on the early years of life dissatisfied Jung who believed that human life involved a continual series of *metamorphoses* or changes in personality orientation through which the process of *individuation* could be achieved.[3] One goal of the individuation process was the unification of personality. Simply stated, Jung viewed the personality as being made up of various psychic components such as the anima and animus (male and female traits) and the shadow (ignored aspects of the self). Although Jung did view old age as a

---

[2]Bühler, "Human Life Goals in the Humanistic Perspective," p. 49.

[3]H. F. Ellenberger, *The Discovery of the Unconscious* (New York: Basic Books, 1970).

period of complete dependence on others, and in some respects as a stage similar to childhood, he had much to say about personality changes specific to old age.[4]

Perhaps the principal contribution made by Jung to the personality of old age was his postulation of changes in the process of psychic organization of the self. This process involved a tendency for the personality to change in the direction of the opposite sex. Thus, he believed that the female component (anima) in older men became more prominent and women became more masculine in their psychological orientation as they aged.

Interestingly, cross-cultural research concerned with age changes in the psychological stances of both men and women seem to uphold Jung's earlier clinically derived notions. Guttman, for example, notes that in contrast to younger men older men are less aggressive, more affiliative, more interested in love than in power, more aesthetic, less businesslike, and more sensitive to the importance of incidental pleasures. He also states that older men turn toward a psychology of "diffuse sensuality," i.e., they become particularly interested in food, pleasant sights, sounds, and human associations. Guttman further reports that studies across a wide range of cultures show that women age psychologically in the reverse direction of men. That is, they become more aggressive, less sentimental, and more domineering in their psychological orientation.[5]

The above results are not related to specific individuals, but they do describe general trends based on group data. However, such sex role changes in psychological orientation might indeed take their toll on married couples in the later stages of life if they do not understand this process.

Although Jung considered the natural end in life to be wisdom and not senility, he believed that the aged individual could only achieve such wisdom by not competing with the youth of society or clinging to the past. Jung appears to have strongly believed that the perpetuation of pseudo-youthful images by the aged in Western societies was deplorable in comparison to the dignity of elders observed in certain anthropological tribal studies.[6] As opposed to clinging to the past or competing with the

---

[4]C. G. Jung, *Memories, Dreams, Reflections* (New York: Pantheon Books, 1963); C. G. Jung, "The Stages of Life," in *The Collected Works of C. G. Jung: Structure and Dynamics of the Psyche*, vol. 8, trans., R. F. C. Hull (New York: Pantheon Books, 1960).

[5]D. Guttman, "Parenthood: A Key to the Comparative Study of the Life Cycle," in *Life-Span Developmental Psychology: Normative Life Crises*, eds., N. Datan and L. H. Ginsberg (New York: Academic Press, 1975).

[6]Ellenberger, *The Discovery of the Unconscious.*

youth of society, Jung maintained that the old person must not deny his current reality and that death should not be "a peril to shrink from ... [for] ... an old man who cannot bid farewell to life appears as feeble and sickly as a young man who is unable to embrace it."[7]

Jung further suggests that as the individual ages he goes through a continuing process of interiorization, i.e., that life psycholgically contracts. The positive aspect of this turn of attention inward is that it enables an inner exploration that may help the person find a meaning and wholeness in his life that makes it possible for him to accept death, Thus, in Jung we see the abstract beginnings of a theory of normal psychological aging which, along with the aforementioned work of Bühler, stresses age-appropriate coping behaviors and tasks. With the work of Erikson, to whom we now turn, we see a slightly more specific approach to the tasks of old age.

Erik Erikson: the resolutions of psychosocial tasks

In a manner similar to Bühler and Jung, Erik Erikson also saw the need to understand the process of personality development throughout the life cycle. Somewhat more specifically than Bühler and Jung, Erikson delineated eight stages of development, each stage representing a psychosocial crisis or task defined by a combination of cultural and maturational needs. The successful resolution of each of these stage-related psychosocial crises is thought to determine the individual's self-evaluation, his success in adapting to both inner psychic and socially imposed tasks, and the future development of his personality. A brief summary of Erikson's eight stages, psychosocial crises, and the psychological quality derived from successful resolution of each crisis is given in Table 3.1.

Although Erikson has stipulated that each of the crises, outlined in Table 3.1, is not necessarily bound to a specific age, he does maintain that there is a strong likelihood for each crisis to be in the foreground at the appropriate stage. He also notes that individuals probably oscillate between two stages at any point in the life cycle and that resolution of earlier crises moderates successful entry into later stages.[8] Table 3.1 shows that the psychosocial crisis most prevalent in old age is integrity versus despair.

---

[7]Jung, "The Stages of Life," p. 20.

[8]E. H. Erikson, "Reflections on Dr. Borg's Life Cycle," *Daedalus* **105** (1976): 1–28.

Table 3.1 Erikson's stages, psychosocial crises, and outcome of successful resolution*

Stage	Psychosocial Crises	Outcome (if resolved)
Infancy	Trust versus mistrust	Hope
Early Childhood	Autonomy versus shame, doubt	Will
Play Age	Initiative versus guilt	Purpose
School Age	Industry versus inferiority	Competence
Adolescence	Identity versus identity confusion	Fidelity
Young Adulthood	Intimacy versus isolation	Love
Maturity	Generativity versus self-absorption	Care
Old Age	Integrity versus despair, disgust	Wisdom

*Adapted from E. H. Erikson, "Reflections on Dr. Borg's Life Cycle," Daedalus 105 (1976): 22.

The conflict between integrity and despair involved the task of reconciling to one's satisfaction that one's life has had purpose and meaning. It involves ". . . the acceptance of one's own and only life cycle and of the people who have become significant to it as something that had to be and that, by necessity, permitted no substitution.[9] The opposite side of the coin is *despair,* the feeling that time is too short for making radical changes in life or that alternate roads are no longer possible. Erikson tells us:

> . . . this is why the elderly try to "doctor" their memories. Rationalized bitterness and disgust can mask that despair, which in severe psychopathology aggravates a senile syndrome of depression, hypochondria, and paranoiac hate. For, whatever chance to transcend the limitations of his self seems to depend on his full (if often tragic) engagement in the one and only life cycle permitted to him.[10]

Erikson goes on to remind us that the task faced by older people is not the total victory of integrity *over* despair and disgust, but rather the achievement of a favorable balance in integrity's favor. According to his formulation, both experiences are inevitable in old age. The experience of despair is there for all old people, no matter how much they have achieved or how much they

[9]E. H. Erikson, "Identity and the Life Cycle," *Psychological Issues* 1 (1959): 98.
[10]Erikson, "Reflections on Dr. Borg's Life Cycle," p. 23.

take on a realistic attitude about life. Erikson's theory, then, implies that those working with the aged should not necessarily encourage the denial of death, but rather the assimilation of its reality into the experience of life—just as integrity should absorb and assimilate the inevitable experiences of despair.

Thus, the appropriate resolution of the conflict of integrity versus despair results in a sense of wisdom, which is "the detached and yet active concern with life itself in the face of death itself, and that it maintains and conveys the integrity of experience, in spite of the decline of bodily and mental functions."[11]

Peck: expansion of Erikson's theory

Although Erikson, as did Bühler and Jung, addressed themselves to issues in personality development in later life, their observations and descriptions might be considered rather global and generalized. In this light, Peck attempted to further delineate and specify the issues that are crucial in old age.[12] Peck also specified what he thought were the crucial issues of middle age as related to issues in later life (see Table 3-2).

Table 3.2 Description and outline of Peck's stages and psychological issues of later life

Stage	Psychological Issue	Description
Middle Age	(a) Valuing wisdom versus valuing physical powers	Successful aging involves the ability to rely on life experience and cognitive abilities, rather than physical strength or stamina. Depression can result if the shift is not made.
	(b) Socializing versus sexualizing in human relationships	Aging persons must reconcile the appearance of the sexual climacteric by allowing the sexual element in their relationships to play a lessened role. New and deeper emphasis on friend-

---

[11]Ibid., p. 23.

[2]R. C. Peck, "Psychological Developments in the Second Half of Life," in *Psychological Aspects of Aging*, ed., J. E. Anderson (Washington, D.C.: American Psychological Association, 1956).

Stage	Psychological Issue	Description
		ship and companionship aspects can potentially improve and strengthen marital and other interpersonal relations.
	(c) Cathectic flexibility versus cathective impoverishment	Cathectic (or emotional) flexibility: the capacity to make new relationships in the face of inevitable losses as children leave home, parents die, and friendship patterns change is crucial for successful aging. Positive adaptation to aging requires the development of a *generalized set* to making new as well as redefining existing emotional relationships (as when children grow up).
	(d) Mental flexibility versus mental rigidity	The ability to remain open to new ideas and to learn from new experiences as opposed to being dominated by a set of inflexible rules "automatically" governing behavior is important for a continuing sense of growth in later life.
Old Age	(a) Ego differentiation versus work-role preoccupation	Successful adaptation to old age may require the establishment of a variety of valued activities and new roles to modify the impact of occupational loss or change in parental and other roles.
	(b) Body transcendence versus body preoccupation	The ability to focus on the comforts and enjoyments of social interactions and mental tasks while deemphasizing body pains and frailties.
	(c) Ego transcendence versus ego preoccupation	Stresses the importance of living as unselfishly and generously as possible in order to insure that one's personal death is not as important in comparison to the awareness that through children, through contributions to the culture, or through one's friendships one's actions will remain significant beyond one's lifetime. Though death is inevitable, human beings can experi-

Stage	Psychological Issue	Description
		ence sense of gratification and meaning for their lives in the future potential of their ideas, family, or future generations of the species.

Adapted from R. C. Peck, "Psychological Developments in the Second Half of Life," in *Psychological Aspects of Aging*, ed., J.E. Anderson (Washington, D.C.: American Psychological Association, 1956), pp. 44–49.

Peck describes middle age as being on a continuum that leads to old age. By comparing polar extremes he offers a model of what may be conceptualized as successful aging compared to nonsuccessful aging, similar to that which we observed in Erikson.

Butler: the life review process

A personality characteristic that many people associate specifically with old age is the phenomenon of reminiscence. Although lay people may attribute this concern for past events shown by older individuals as escape from the present or as senility, it has been pointed out that reminiscence may serve a number of useful functions in the psychological organization of the aged. For example, Butler, a research psychiatrist, has theorized that reminiscence is part of a normal and healthy *life review process* brought about by the realization of the closeness of death.[13] Manifestations of the life review include mirror gazing, nostalgia, interests in story telling, reconsideration of past activities, and flashes of extreme clarity about early life events. During the life review it is not uncommon for some older people to "spill out" their life story to anyone who will listen while other older people may speak in a monologue without apparent concern for the presence or absence of others.[14] Thus, it is advised that those who work with the aged train themselves to listen thoughtfully instead of ignore the reminiscences of older people for reminiscence may serve a therapeutic function.

---

[13]R. M. Butler, "Re-awakening Interest," *Nursing Homes* 10 (1961): 8–19.

[14]R. M. Butler and M. I. Lewis, *Aging and Mental Health* (St. Louis: Mosby Publishers, 1973).

It should be stressed that the life review will probably lead to some negative feelings and regrets. In its more severe forms, it can lead to feelings of depression, anxiety, guilt, despair, and obsessional ruminations about past mistakes. On balance, however, the life review can for many people (especially if they had been fairly integrated in earlier life) yield positive results, such as healing old disputes with enemies, attempting to right old wrongs, correcting any changes in negative attitudes toward relatives or friends, engendering a sense of pride in one's achievements, and culminating a feeling of personal serenity—perhaps related to the belief that one has done his best in life. It might also be noted that such creative works as memoirs, scrapbooks, family albums, and other interests kindled in old age may be the results of the life review. For these latter reasons, the sensitive worker should encourage this process if in his judgment it appears beneficial.

Kübler-Ross: personality organization and the process of dying

It is only in recent history that specific attempts have been made to understand whether there are psychologically "normal" styles of responding to the harsh reality of death. One of the more sensitive attempts to understand personality changes in the terminally ill was carried out by Kübler-Ross, a psychiatrist and researcher who interviewed a large number of dying patients and who has developed a stage theory of the dying process.[15] Kübler-Ross's theory proposes that the process of dying normally consists of an orderly progression of five adaptive stages. Although Kübler-Ross assumes that these stages follow one another in a sequential order, others have noted that individuals can be observed to oscillate among all or some of the stages every few hours.[16] Thus, we believe it is more helpful to consider the following five stages as distinguishable but not necessarily sequential crises periods in the dying process. The five stages are described below.[17]

Denial and isolation. The initial response to the awareness of death may be a temporary state of shock and numbness followed by

[15]E. Kübler-Ross, *On Death and Dying* (New York: The Macmillan Company, 1969).

[16]R. Kastenbaum, "Is Death a Life Crisis?" in *Life-Span Developmental Psychology: Normative Life Crises*, eds., Datan and Ginsberg.

[17]Kübler-Ross, *On Death and Dying*.

the feeling that it "must be a mistake." The vast majority of patients interviewed by Kübler-Ross held onto their need for denial for relatively short periods; only 3 of 200 interviewed held onto this denial to the very last.

This initial defensive process is seen as beneficial because it gives the patient time to develop less stringent defenses to cope with the reality of his situation. It is suggested that this initial denial should be respected as a normal and healthy process of coping with unpleasant and shocking news. Those who work with the terminally ill (e.g., nurses, etc.) should not attempt to prematurely discuss their patient's feelings. It is suggested that the patient himself will reveal his willingness to deal with the issue of death when he acknowledges the reality of his own situation.

Although premature discouragement of denial is not useful, Kübler-Ross also notes that hospital workers, who for their own personality reasons feel the need to deny the patient's death, may encourage their patients to maintain a pretense of well-being. It is also suggested that the sensitive worker should expect terminal patients who have gone beyond this stage to occasionally, and throughout their illness, momentarily isolate the reality of their impending death from awareness.

Anger. As the patient's denial of his impending death diminishes, a new feeling of anger, envy, and resentment best summarized as "why me" emerges. No one is exempt from this anger for the patient seems to be struggling to blame somebody for this overwhelming disaster. Often hospital personnel, relatives, and friends may become targets for this anger. Kübler-Ross advises that it is crucial for those who work with or visit the dying to recognize the symptoms of the *anger stage* and not take it personally. She observes that staff or family who react personally may tend to curtail visits and otherwise avoid the patient who, in reality, needs their attention and care. Anger must be recognized as the beginning of an acceptance of the reality of one's death.

Bargaining. Once the anger stage subsides, many terminally ill patients can be observed to engage in forms of bargaining patterns. It is as if the person is trying to make a deal with fate by changing his strategy from one of anger to asking for a favor. Kübler-Ross sees this behavior as similar to the maneuver of the child who turns the anger of having been denied permission by parents to visit a friend overnight into the query, "If I am very good all week and wash the dishes every evening, then will you let me go?" It is in this manner that many terminally ill patients attempt to gain postponements, often by making secretive deals with God. Kübler-Ross suggests that some bargains may be expressions of long-standing unresolved guilt, such as offerings to be righteous or to do church work, and might usefully be resolved by staff if so recognized.

Depression. Eventually, the terminally ill patient becomes depressed. This experience may be precipitated by the need for further surgery, more symptoms, or physical changes caused by the illness. In effect, denial, anger, and bargaining become replaced with a sense of great loss. Kübler-Ross notes that two kinds of depressions may be observed: a *reactive depression* and a *preparatory depression.* Reactive depression may be identified as the sense of shame and sadness that results from the removal of valued physical features (such as that experienced by a woman whose uterus or breast was removed because of cancer). Preparatory depression involves a sense of sadness precipitated by the realization of impending losses due to one's death. Both forms of depression should be identified and dealt with in different ways. Reactive depression may be dealt with by directly attempting to enhance the patient's self-esteem, such as providing a breast prosthesis for the breast cancer victim or complimenting a woman for some especially feminine feature if it is known that she no longer feels like a "woman" because of her surgery. In these situations good cheer and frequent visiting may be of some help. Preparatory depression should not, according to Kübler-Ross, be dealt with by direct attempts to cheer the patient up. Encouragements and reassurances are not as meaningful for patients in this phase. Instead, Kübler-Ross suggests that the patient be allowed to fully express his sorrow. Often silently sitting with the patient and quietly interacting by touching or holding his hand (just "being with" the patient) may be sufficient to help him gain a personal acceptance of his impending death.

Acceptance. If death has not been sudden or unexpected and if the patient has had sufficient time to work through the first four stages, he will reach the stage of acceptance. During this final stage the patient seems "almost void of feelings." Tired and weak, the patient senses that the "struggle" is over and that the time for the final rest before the long journey has come. It is during this stage that the family may need more attention and support than the dying patient does. In part, they may not understand that the patient may wish to be left alone much of the time or does not feel talkative in the presence of even the closest family members. Again, as in the preparatory depression phase, it is recommended that quiet, empathetic, silent communication such as holding the patient's hand is all the patient really desires.

In discussing the foregoing five stages of the normal ways of coping with death, Kübler-Ross elucidates some important guidelines for those who work with the terminally ill and aged. She clearly demystifies the last stage of her life for family members and friends of dying patients. Her general sensitivity to the topic leads her to one final insight, i.e., the notion that the phenomenon of *hope* is underneath it all, stabilizing the dying patient's ability to live through the weeks and months of suffering. Most importantly, she also suggests that staff, by reinforcing this notion, can aid the patient in this normal and healthy process.

Her general sensitivity to the topic is remarkable and her outline of what to recognize is as humanistic as it is practical. However, we must also insert a note of caution about her theory and its implications for practical use.[18] Researchers, for example, have noted that her theory is not yet a proven fact or empirically demonstrated but, rather, it stands as a significant clinical report of the personal experiences with dying patients by essentially one observer. A second criticism of the theory is that it does not take into account potential differences between males and females. For example, it appears that women may be more upset by the impact of their death on others while males may feel more concerned with loss of stature of power. It also has been pointed out that the nature of the disease, the ethnicity of the patient, the lifelong personality or cognitive styles of the patient, as well as the environment in which the person is dying (i.e., an alienating nursing home or the same house in which the person was born, etc.) must be taken into account.

Perhaps the most important criticism of practical significance is the notion that those who work with the aged should be careful to distinguish between what usually happens and what the theory says *should* happen during the dying process. Kübler-Ross herself cautioned that dying patients should not be *rushed* through the various stages. Thus, as with any theory, we suggest that the Kübler-Ross stages be viewed as useful guidelines through which we may gain an increased understanding of the normal changes in psychological orientation to be expected in the last phase of life.

---

[18]Kastenbaum, "Is Death a Life Crisis?"

The Cultural Context of the Aging Process

Previously we discussed the biological processes and aspects of
normal personality development in old age. In order to more fully
understand the complex of forces that influences who the aged are,
we must focus on the cultural context in which the aged live. What
does society expect old people to be like? What are these
expectations based on and what implications do these expectations
have for the problems encountered by those who work with the
aged? It is to these and related issues that we now turn.

cultural definitions

The criteria for defining old age vary from society to society.
In many simple cultures old age is defined in functional terms, i.e.,
at the point where biological deterioration literally prevents the
individual from carrying out his traditional work or other valuable
role functions. In these societies the old are "the about to die," not
those who have reached some particular chronological age. This
definition of old age is very different from the formal
chronological one that typifies American society.[19] In American
society old age begins at age 65. Many people do not seem to realize
that this criterion is purely cultural and is a definition originally
based on the traditional start of eligibility for social security
benefits.

We might suspect that as the retirement age changes, the
cultural definitions of when old age begins will also change. Early
retirement, however (whether brought about by affluence or
planned unemployment), may pose new problems for those who
need to discover meaningful substitute activities. The importance
of the foregoing issue is heightened by recent estimates that
indicate that the average member of society will soon spend more
than half his or her life outside the labor force.[20] Indeed, the
setting of progressively earlier retirement ages in combination with
the phenomenon of increasing longevity will probably cause a

---

[19]M. Clark, "The Anthropology of Aging: A New Area for Studies of Culture and
Personality," in *Middle Age and Aging*, ed., B. L. Neugarten (Chicago: The University of
Chicago Press, 1968).

[20]J. E. Birron and D. S. Woodruff, "Human Development over the Life Span through
Education," in *Life Span Developmental Psychology: Personality and Socialization*, eds., P. B.
Baltes and K. W. Schaie (New York: Academic Press, 1973).

series of socially induced psychological problems; our society may be creating a new life stage that contains no specific role definitions for the aged. The problem is further compounded by the cultural tendency of Americans to downgrade nonwork or leisure activities upon retirement.[21]

roles and norms

The concept of social role is an important one for the understanding of the position of the aged in our society. For present purposes, a *role* may be defined as a content area within a social system that has specific action characteristics. For example, the role of mother, father, truck driver, student, wife, etc., are reasonably identifiable content areas within our American social system that carry with them specific kinds of behaviors (or action characteristics) that are readily predictable. Most people, for example, if asked to playact a "student" or "truck driver" could do so without having to know much about the individual personality characteristics, i.e., all students study or read or sit in classes, etc. That certain roles are predictable and the behaviors they imply very specific can also be seen by the fact that we can quickly identify someone who performs outside his appropriate role, for example, the 75-year-old woman who wears a bikini or the 80-year-old man who develops an interest in sky diving.

These examples may be construed to indicate that certain roles are probably considered inappropriate for an elderly person in terms of current social norms. It is not "right" to show off one's body or engage in dangerous sports unless one is young and/or has a certain physical build. Role behaviors, then, are governed by normative prescriptions, i.e., what we should be doing as fathers, mothers, men, women, students, etc. The development, acceptance, and internalization of these "shoulds" may be called the process of socialization. It is through this process, which involves exposure to parents, the educational system, the mass media, peer pressures, etc., that one learns to perform particular roles in terms of the social norms of any given society. It is only when a society does not socialize the individual for appropriate roles or has not as yet defined the appropriate roles (as may be the case for long periods of retirement and old age in the United States) that problems in adjustment may ensue.

---

[21]R. J. Havighurst, "Social Roles, Work, Leisure, and Education," in *The Psychology of Adult Development and Aging,* eds., C. Eisdorfer and M. P. Lawton (Washington, D.C.: American Psychological Association, 1973).

We should also be aware that societies vary greatly in terms of
the roles and norms for which they socialize their participants.
Thus, when an individual learns one set of norms and roles but
then emigrates to a new and different society, he may have great
difficulty in adjusting and may be considered deviant or even
mentally ill. Psychiatrists and psychologists, for example,
sometimes encounter problems in diagnosing the adjustment of
foreign-born or recently arrived elderly who believe in
spiritualism. To these aged, hearing and seeing spirits and
experiencing visitations may be very normal and related to roles
learned in their previous cultural settings. It would seem to be of
great importance that those who work with the aged be aware of
the possibility that behavior in the elderly that may appear bizarre
or deviant by current norms may be the product of the anticipation
of aging in another culture or the results of values learned in
another time period in history.

age grading and anticipatory socialization

Age grading refers to the notion that all societies organize the
life span into stages or time periods during which an individual is
expected to do certain things (e.g., attend school, marry, work,
retire, and even to die) or to behave in certain ways (e.g., play in
childhood, be achievement-oriented in youth, and nonsexual in
old age). Age grades are chronological aspects of social norms.
There have been some indications that age grading can pose a
great problem for the aged in our society. For example, in a study
of mentally well and mentally ill elderly, Clark found that the value
orientations considered healthy for younger and middle-aged
people were often associated with mental illness in old age.[22] She
noted that those elderly diagnosed as mentally ill seemed to cling to
precisely those patterns of value orientation upheld as most
representative of the core values and norms of American society in
the years they had been middle-aged persons, i.e., the values and
norms of individualism, competitiveness, aggressiveness,
acquisitiveness of money, future orientation, etc. Clark implies that
mental illness in old age may inolve an inability to give up
previously held values and move into the next age grade. She
concludes that normal aging in our society depends on the

---

[22]Clark, "The Anthropology of Aging: A New Area for Studies of Culture and
Personality."

acceptance of a culturally prescribed value shift (or age grade) imposed upon those entering old age status.

Age grading may also serve useful purposes, especially if we think of its role in the process of anticipatory socialization. Anticipatory socialization is the process of preparing for a change in role or status. It involves the ability, and time, to explore and try out new norms or expectations that will be associated with a new role or status once the change is made.

Simple societies, for example, tend to provide ample opportunity for anticipatory socialization. The close interaction with the elders in the small populations of these societies provides an opportunity to model, identify, and become familiar with the roles and norms characteristic of the aged. Since in these societies the average longevity is low, the ratio of elders to the available "job slots" and ceremonial positions is also low. Because of these factors, the middle aged in simple societies often have "something" they can actually look forward to doing, or being, when they reach old age. Thus, many anthropological studies have found a positive correlation between the existence of age grades and the continuation into important political, religious, or ceremonial offices of aged men.[23]

Unlike what occurs in many tribal societies in which the young member knows that he will inevitably accede to the status of leader—if he survives—American society does not seem to provide a set of clearly defined role expectations and norms for the elderly. If we also note that American society has more people who live longer per capita than do most tribal groups (because of improved child care, etc.), we can see that complete anticipatory socialization may be at best a difficult task for the young and middle-aged generations. The task of discovering new roles for old age is further complicated by the high value placed on individual development and freedom of action in the United States.

Some social scientists have noted that at least for the urban, affluent aged, a new set of norms involving the general value of activity as opposed to work is becoming institutionalized.[24] Upon retirement, leisure, "as long as it is marked by some activity, has become a value in American life."[25] It seems that as long as

---

[23]M. Clark, "An Anthropological View of Retirement," in *Retirement,* ed., F. M. Carp (New York: Behavioral Publications, 1972).

[24]S. J. Miller, "The Social Dilemma of the Aging Leisure Participant," in *Middle Age and Aging,* ed., Neugarten; Clark, "An Anthropological View of Retirement."

[25]Clark, "An Anthropological View of Retirement."

Americans are "doing something" or "keeping busy" they may feel useful and worthwhile. In this light, it is relevant to note that the trend toward age-segregated retirement communities where affluent elderly may pursue active lives, independent of their children, may become a new norm for which anticipatory socialization is to be inaugurated. The cost for such a norm may be very high in the sense that it perpetuates the physical and psychological separation of the older and younger generations and may, in the long run, be very detrimental to the future of our social organization. Further, such a norm does not solve the problems encountered by the poor or economically deprived elderly—who make up a substantial proportion of our population.

Thus, although age grading may be beneficial because it helps the elderly through the process of anticipatory socialization to become familiar and accept their new status, the American version may be ultimately dysfunctional in that anticipatory socialization involves age segregation that encourages separateness between the generations. These factors must be kept in mind by all those who work with the aged.

attitudes toward aging

A major impact of the socialization process in any society involves its effect on the formation of attitudes toward aging and the aged. If American society most clearly emphasizes the value of norms and roles relevant to work and achievement orientation, so that people are valued for their utility instead of their worth, then we might expect that most people would not look forward to growing old. We might also note that the kinds of feelings toward aging that are engendered by society may have critical effects on the capacity of people to adjust or even survive in old age. For example, Bennett and Eckman noted that those elderly who have negative attitudes toward their own aging may lack the motivation to seek needed services, health care, or other assistance. In addition, the old people's negative attitudes toward aging may alienate younger members of the community and increase the gap between age groups.[26] Positive attitudes, however, might engender understanding and empathy for a life stage that most Americans will live to experience. In this light, we turn to a brief survey of

---

[26]R. Bennett and J. Eckman, "Attitudes Toward Aging: A Critical Examination of Recent Literature and Implications for Future Research," in *The Psychology of Adult Development and Aging*, eds., Eisdorfer and Lawton.

research done on attitudes toward aging among various age groups, including the aged themselves.

Among the first to study attitudes toward aging were Tuckman and Lorge. They developed a simple questionnaire that presumably tapped negative stereotypes and misconceptions about various aspects of aging. Their questionnaire consisted of statements about old people (to which respondents answered either yes or no), such as: "Old people need glasses to read." "They are in the happiest period of their lives." "They get upset easily." "They just like to sit and dream."[27]

In general, research on the Tuckman and Lorge questionnaire supports the view that old people are devalued by both young and old respondents. One interesting study that used a modified version of the Tuckman-Lorge questionnaire was carried out by Axelrod and Eisdorfer. They asked a sample of college students to give their opinions on the Tuckman-Lorge items as they related to five different age categories: 35, 45, 55, 65, and 75. The results showed that the ascription of negative attitudes by the young people increased for each decade from 35 to 75 years.[28]

A slightly different approach used to tap attitudes toward old people consists of sentence-completion tests.[29] This approach involves the presentation of short sentence stems such as: "In general old people need . . ." which respondents then complete in any manner they wish. Research using the sentence-completion format shows that the young and the old may indeed differ in their attitudes and beliefs about old age and old people. Some examples of the way different age groups have responded to the sentence completion method are given below.

One of the greatest fears of many old people is . . . . Younger respondents tended to consider "death or dying" as the greatest fear. Older people stressed "lack of money" and "financial insecurity." In analyzing this response the authors suggest that closeness to death may not necessarily imply an increase of fear of death at the conscious level. They speculate that a denial process may be at work among the older respondents. They also note that the differences between old and young respondents on this

---

[27]J. Tuckman and I. Lorge, "Attitudes Toward Old People," *Journal of Social Psychology* **37** (1953): 249–260.

[28]S. Axelrod and C. Eisdorfer, "Attitudes Toward Old People: An Empirical Analysis of the Stimulous Group Validity of the Tuckman–Lorge Questionnaire," *Journal of Gerontology* **16** (1961): 75–80.

[29]N. Kogan and F. C. Shelton, "Beliefs About 'Old People': A Comparative Study of Older and Younger Samples," *The Journal of Genetic Psychology* **100** (1962): 93–111.

question point out the existence of cross-generational differences
in understanding the problems of the aged.

Old people tend to resent . . . . Kogan and Shelton found that the
young respondents tended to cite themselves or the general
category of "younger people" as the object of old people's
resentments. Older respondents were more specific in their
answers, referring to "rejection," "lack of concern," and "reference
to age." The authors suggest that the old people were somewhat
concerned (at least implicitly) with the attitudes of the young
toward them.

In summarizing their research, Kogan and Shelton imply that
old people may be somewhat defensive about how others see them,
that they probably try to anticipate the feelings of the younger
generation in order to gain acceptance, and that they try to avoid
the possibility of rejection by that dominant majority. Ineed, as we
shall subsequently note, this socially induced defensiveness on the
part of old people may be the cause of the observed high degree of
cautiousness among the aged, a cautiousness that may have
erroneously been interpreted as evidence that the old lack the
ability to do certain tasks.

▸ the culture of caution

The belief that old people are more conservative in their
approach to life than are their younger counterparts and the
notion of a generation gap of caution seem to have been accepted
by social scientists for many decades. In fact, the popular belief that
the aged are uncomfortable with the new and the uncertain, expect
failure, fear rejection, have a low degree of self-confidence, and
avoid obtaining information about their abilities has been
documented by the research literature.[30] We shall now turn to
some of the research evidence and then comment on the possibility
that cultural factors might explain much of the need for certainty
and low risk taking evidenced by the aged.

Errors of omission.   As a group, the aged are more likely to
commit errors of omission instead of errors of commission. An
error of omission involves a nonresponse (not answering a
question on a test). An error of commission involves making a

---

[30]M. A. Okum and F. J. Divesta, "Cautiousness in Adulthood as a Function of Age and
Instructions," *Journal of Gerontology* **31** (1976): 571–576; J. Botwinick, *Aging and Behavior*
(New York: Springer, 1973).

mistake (for example, providing the wrong answer on a test or making a wrong decision instead of not deciding). The omission error may stem from a desire for certainty, as a way of avoiding failure and maximizing self-esteem. The virtue of this is that old people have a tendency to make few mistakes on tasks if given sufficient time.[31] As a consequence, many elderly do not do well on intelligence tests because many of the tests require answers within specific time limits.

- *Risk taking.* The tendency toward caution among the aged seems to exist not only where abilities or capacities are at issue but also where choices, preferences, or behavior are called for. For example, Wallach and Kogan found that old people were considerably more cautious than the young (especially in making decisions involving financial matters) on a risk-taking questionnaire they constructed.[32] This questionnaire consisted of 12 different "everyday life situations" involving dilemmas of choice. Each situation described a central person who is supposed to choose between two courses of action. One course in each situation was very risky but involved the possibility of considerable gain if successful. Each young or old respondent was faced with the task of "advising" the person in each of the 12 situations on what degree of certainty he should require before choosing the risky alternative. The choices range from 10 percent certainty (i.e., great risk) to 90 percent certainty (i.e., low risk). Respondents also had the option of choosing the most conservative alternative, that is, making *no* decision to follow the risky course of action. An example of one such choice dilemma follows:

> Mr. A., an electrical engineer who is married and has one child, has been working for a large electronics corporation since graduating from college five years ago. He is assured of a lifetime job with a modest, though adequate salary, and liberal pension benefits upon retirement. On the other hand, it is very unlikely that his salary will increase much before he retires. While attending a convention, Mr. A. is offered a job with a small, newly founded company with a highly uncertain future. The new job would pay more to start and would offer the possibility of a share in the ownership if the company survived the competition of the larger firms.[33]

[31]J. Botwinick, *Aging and Behavior.*

[32]M. Wallach and N. Kogan, "Aspects of Judgment and Decision Making: Interrelations and Changes with Age," *Behavioral Science* **6** (1961): 23–36.

[33]Ibid., p. 27.

Respondents are asked to select the lowest probability they would consider to make it worthwhile to "advise" Mr. A. to take the new job (or to advise that no decision be taken).

The Wallach-Kogan items have been criticized for not being totally relevant to the aged and have since been modified by Botwinick.[34] Botwinick also found that the elderly were more cautious in their approach to risky decisions than were the younger people.

We could leave this section by stating that indeed the elderly are more cautious. This is not the complete story, however, especially for those who intend to work with the aged. You may recall that the original Wallach–Kogan items allowed the respondent to choose a no-risk alternative (i.e., to advise not taking the new job in the case of Mr. A., etc.). Botwinick's items also contained this option. Further analysis of his results showed that the elderly have a very strong tendency to choose this no-risk alternative. What does this mean in terms of decision-making processes in the aged? What happens when older subjects are not given the option to choose a no-risk alternative? Although we might logically expect that they would then opt for the next most conservative choices available, i.e., 90 percent certainty, this is, in fact, not the case. When a new questionnaire compelled both young and old respondents to take *some* degree of risk, age differences in cautiousness were not seen at all.[35]

Thus, when risk cannot be avoided, we see that old people may be as venturesome as their younger counterparts. The only time they seem to be cautious (at least in experimental settings) is when this caution is a permissible alternative. Thus, old people may not really be reluctant to be somewhat risky (or venturesome) if the situation demands it. What seems to be required is that the situation be specifically structured to enable old people to function in this capacity. However, many situations in life do not involve clearly structured demands or activities. One exception is certain aspects of the world of work, and as we have seen the aged are virtually excluded from this world as a function of the social security and automatic retirement laws. This only leaves the area of leisure for many of the aged. Leisure, however, is unstructured time, a domain of experience in which we have opportunity to

---

[34]J. Botwinick, "Cautiousness in Advanced Age," *Journal of Gerontology* **21** (1966): 347–353.

[35]J. Botwinick, "Disinclination to Venture Response Versus Cautiousness in Responding," *Journal of Genetic Psychology* **115** (1969): 55–62.

exercise maximal choice.[36] Leisure settings may thus not afford the demands to be venturesome that some old people might need.

In light of the above, Brok and Westcott studied the free time preferences of individuals in adolescence, young adulthood, adulthood, and old age.[37] When asked to choose from a list of options, the way they preferred to spend their free time, older people preferred activities involving a great deal of order and pre-planning. This was the opposite of younger respondents who least preferred such activities. The younger and adult groups most preferred activities involving social affiliation and private autonomy needs. The high preference shown for "order" by the older people in the above study might be indicative of the tendency (when given the option) for the aged to feel more comfortable about time they can structure and control—perhaps in a way analogous to the low risk findings previously discussed.

But if the elderly are really not that cautious in situations that prevent them from exercising the cautious option, we still need to explain why they choose the certain, more conservative road whenever possible. One explanation favored by the present authors involves the values and socialization effects of American society. Our culture is oriented toward the young and there seem to be few healthy norms available to the old. One of the few norms in existence may be reflected by the attitude and risk studies cited above. Indeed, perhaps there is a norm of caution, socially induced and culturally backed, which society expects the elderly individual to adhere to almost magically upon retirement. The probability that such traits are socially influenced as opposed to being strictly of a biological nature is evident from the fact that if called upon, the aged do show the same risk-taking tendencies of the young. This, of course, is not to say that there are no real changes with age. Rather, it seems that the elderly act as they are expected to, but when they do they are devalued by the young who live by a different set of values. This then becomes a self-fulfilling prophecy. What is expected of the old is seen as confirmed when the old conform, and then their conformity is devalued.

Could it be "that there may well be a conspiracy on the part of the middle aged to remove the old from active participation in

---

[36] A. J. Brok, "Issues in Leisure Relevant to Counseling and Applied Human Development," paper presented at the 83rd annual meeting of the American Psychological Association, Chicago, 1975.

[37] A. J. Brok and N. Westcott, "Age and Sex Differences in Free Time Interests: An Exploratory Inquiry," paper presented at the 46th annual meeting of the Eastern Psychological Association, New York, 1975.

society"?[38] For example, it has been suggested that some deficits observed in intelligence tests given to the aged are the result of the effects of socially induced policies. As Schaie notes:

> . . . at least some older people do less well when they are afraid of involvement in a task involving unreasonable risk of loss or embarrassment, but that careful control of instructional set may well induce the older person to consider alternatives he might otherwise eschew.[39]

Schaie suggests that one solution to the dilemma of the old is for workers in the field to use the knowledge that the aged will show a normal predilection toward risk taking if given no choice in the matter. For example, compulsory education requirements might be set up for older populations (as they are for younger) or alternatively adequate reinforcements or reward contingencies could be made available for voluntary participation in educational programs. These latter suggestions imply that structured or "moderately challenging" incentives might be used as a way to motivate many of the aged to counteract the detrimental effects of culturally induced cautiousness.

The Environment of the Aged

It may be fairly stated that all human behavior is influenced by the environmental context in which it occurs as well as by individual, biological, and psychological factors. It is only through comprehension of the physical, social, and interpersonal influences that exist "outside" the person and the interaction of these influences with the unique characteristics of any particular person that we can begin to understand human behavior. We also know that as people age, environmental factors seem to play a role of increasing importance on their behavior. In part, the stronger influence of environmental factors among the elderly results from not only their lowered ability to cope with socially induced stress but also from decreases in their physiological competence.[40] Thus,

---

[38]K. W. Schaie, "Translations in Gerontology from Lab to Life: Intellectual Functioning," *American Psychologist* **29** (1974): 802–807 (805).

[39]Ibid., p. 804.

[40]L. Gottesman, C. E. Quarterman, and G. M. Cohn, "Psychosocial Treatment of the Aged," in *The Psychology of Adult Development and Aging,* eds., Eisdorfer and Lawton; L. Nahemow and M. P. Lawton, "Toward an Ecological Theory of Adaptation and Aging," in *Environmental Psychology,* 2nd ed., eds., H. Proshansky, W. H. Ittelson, and L. G. Rivlin (New York: Holt, Rinehart, & Winston, 1976).

it seems clear that those who work with the aged must learn to pay particular attention to the impact of environmental factors. It is to some of these factors that we now shall turn.

living arrangements

In general, living arrangements of the elderly vary from residential single-family houses to the highly institutionalized nursing homes. Between these two extremes there are a number of other options for living that are becoming increasingly important. For example, many older people reside in mobile home parks, which are less expensive than houses but retain some measure of privacy and a sense of independence. Others, especially in the middle- and upper-income groups, turn to retirement villages. In urban areas, housing projects and retirement hotels, often of varying quality, are important residential sites.

It is a misconception that the majority of the elderly live in some form of institution. Recent studies, for example, show that 70 percent of individuals over age 65 actually own their own homes.[41] Unfortunately, those who are homeowners are not exempt from the considerable economic stresses faced by all the elderly, who on average fall among the lowest income groups in the United States. For example, the repair costs, utility bills, and high property taxes involved in maintaining a private dwelling may become major environmental stressors which, in turn, may cause maladaptive coping patterns. Some elderly, for example, attempt to compromise by purchasing less food in order to maintain repair costs or rents. Many are forced to move to or remain in substandard housing which, in turn, creates a spiral of despair and withdrawal. It has been suggested that economic stresses in general can lead to a lowered sense of self-esteem and depression in some of the aged.[42]

age segregation

The question of whether it is better for older people to live in an environment that separates them from other age groups instead of living in age-integrated settings remains unclear. Age-integrated settings, which provide physical proximity between young and old,

---

[41]E. H. Steinfeld, "Ecology of Aging," in *An Instructor's Handbook for the Development of a Basic Course in Gerontology* (Syracuse, N.Y.: Syracuse University All-University Gerontology Center, 1975).

[42]Gottesman, Quarterman, and Cohn, "Psychosocial Treatment of the Aged."

do not necessarily guarantee that the two age groups will relate
socially. The evidence that cross-generational friendships are
encouraged by having different age groups live in close proximity
is very weak.[43] In comparison, age-segregated living
arrangements, particuarly in secure and well-managed apartment
buildings or projects, appear to encourage social interaction
among elderly tenants, especially among those who live on the
same floor.[44]

Although age segregation may be beneficial because it
encourages interaction and provides a degree of peer security
among the elderly, it may be philosophically negative to perpetuate
such living arrangements. Unfortunately, the continued
separation of age groups in our society may only increase and
reinforce the overwhelmingly negative stereotypes and lack of
knowledge the young have about old age. One solution to this
dilemma might be to establish multi-aged community centers in
areas of age-segregated housing. Such centers might serve as
common meeting grounds through which the old and the young
could interact, while not necessarily living in the same housing.

mobility
and the built environment

A brief stroll through most urban and suburban areas in the
United States quickly leads one to the realization that the physical
environment is designed for the active adult, not for small children
or the handicapped and especially not for the aged. It is as if
the elderly had been "vetoed out" of society by architects and
designers.[45] Environmental design features such as steep steps to
subway or commuter trains, inadequately lighted street signs,
traffic lights that change rapidly (thus not giving some older people
sufficient time to cross the street), and insufficient or expensive
public transportation are all factors that can affect the mobility and
exploratory desires of older people. One study, for example,
found that New York urban elderly rarely left their immediate
neighborhood and that they lived within a constricted social
space.[46]

---

[43]Steinfeld, "Ecology of Aging."

[44]W. H. Ittelson, M. H. Proshansky, L. G. Rivlin, and G. H. Winkel, *An Introduction to Environmental Psychology* (New York: Holt, Rinehart, & Winston, 1974).

[45]Ibid.

[46]L. Nahemow and L. S. Kogan, *Reduced Fare for the Elderly* (New York: Mayor's Office for the Aging, 1971).

prosthetic environments

A prosthetic device is an artificial part, such as a limb, etc., which may help an individual function. As applied to environments, it suggests that the aged may be helped to function by proper design features. The concept of a prosthetic environment for the elderly has been discussed in terms of the following categories:[47]

1. *Life-maintenance activity.* This category stresses the importance of physical safety, such as nonskid floors in a house.
2. *Perceptual behavior.* Lawton notes that the use of bright colors can enhance orientation to place as well as overcome the depressive "esthetic barrenness" of some institutional environments. It is also suggested that poor eyesight suffered by many of the elderly can be compensated for by the use of large-faced clocks.
3. *Cognitive behavior.* Room doors (and floors) that are color coded to demarcate important routes (within institutions or elsewhere) help older people "map out" their environment.
4. *Self-maintenance skills.* Bathroom facilities can be arranged to anticipate the physical limits of old age (such as side-bar to hold onto instead of relying on an attendant or helping person to assist with certain toilet functions). Kitchen facilities can be designed for simple nontaxing use by individuals.
5. *Effectance behavior.* The availability of hobbies, various other recreational activities, and "unprogrammed thinking" can enhance morale. However, stress on too active participation is not necessarily optimal. (Lawton notes that much effectance behavior is of the vicarious kind.) Enjoyment is obtained through sitting and watching other more active people.

Additional prosthetic features of especial importance for institutional environments include: (1) *Prosthesis for a sense of time,*

---

[47]M. P. Lawton, "Social and Structural Aspects of Prosthetic Environments for Older People," paper presented at the Third Annual Institute on Man's Adjustment in a Complex Environment, Veterans Administration Hospital, Brecksville, Ohio, June, 1968; M. P. Lawton, "Some Beginnings of an Ecological Psychology of Old Age," in *Environment and the Social Sciences: Perspective and Applications,* eds., J. F. Wohwill and D. H. Caison (Washington, D.C.: American Psychological Association, 1972).

such as numerous and large calendars that clearly show the day, week, or season or that announce important social events, etc. (2) *Prosthesis that enhance the sense of self* as evidenced by the provision of mirrors for client rooms and ample space to store personal objects and display family photographs, pictures, etc. (3) *Prosthesis that encourage staff–patient intermingling.* This can be simply placing staff offices adjoining patient space. (4) *Prosthesis for vicarious social involvement.* This can be arranged by designing nursing homes and other institutions so that ward activity can be easily observed when people sit outside their rooms. This could be done by organizing client rooms in a semicircle around a central activity space. (5) *Prosthesis for autonomy.* It is suggested that nursing home residents should be able to choose different ways of using their environment. This could be done by providing sufficient individual rooms for privacy while also providing space for small groups of residents to sit outside their room doors and converse. (6) *Prosthesis for general social interaction.* One of many suggestions is to design institutions so that corridors intersect. It is assumed that the probability of social interaction increases where pathways of locomotion cross.

optimal environments and the "best fit" idea

In keeping with the notion that human behavior is best understood as the product of the interaction between environmental forces and the unique characteristics of the individual, we must note that all people will not find the same environment as beneficial to their growth, development, or general functioning. The stimulating urban environment that the physically able old person might enjoy exploring may be overwhelmingly stressful to his less physically competent peer. Institutional living that maximizes prosthetic design features may be perfect for some old people, but it may be terribly stifling or dulling for others. The active older person who maintains a strong sense of inner resourcefulness may only need to be informed about activities available in his community in order to become a participant; but the aged individual who stresses the significance of fate, luck, or the influence of others, as opposed to his own sense of initiative, may need to be motivated by an outreach worker if he is to become involved in some community activity. Education or information about "what is out there" may not be sufficient motivation to conquer his fears of traveling to even the safest locations. In sum, the beneficial qualities of any particular environment depend on the psychological and constitutional characteristics of the individual it contains.

Perhaps the best statement on the subject has been made by Nahemow and Lawton who note that the individual functions best when he is in a "moderately challenging environment."[48] They suggest that too much stimulation may be overwhelming and may lead to dysfunctional behavior such as withdrawal but too little stimulation is not challenging enough and can induce lethargy and encourage people to operate below their capacities. The moderately challenging environment is one that *best fits* the optimal functioning capacity of the person. However, we must always keep in mind that what is moderately challenging for one older person may not be so for another. Therefore, those who work with the aged must take into consideration both the capacities of the individual and the challenge provided by the environment. Such thinking can lead to better design of activities and programs for the aged.

Social Characteristics of the Aged

Who are the aged is defined not only by biological processes, aspects of personality development, or cultural and environmental factors, but also by various social characteristics such as population distribution, income and educational levels, and living arrangements. In this section we shall briefly survey some of these social characteristics of aging.

demographics

It has been estimated that there are some 31 million people age 60 years and older in the United States; those age 65 and over number some 22 million. Indications are that this sizeable and diverse group of people is growing both in number and in relative proportion to the rest of the population. For example, the proportion of the United States population that was 60 years and over increased from 14.1 percent in 1970 to 14.7 percent in 1974 while the 65-year-old-and-over group increased from 9.8 percent to 10.3 percent during the same 4-year period. It is estimated that by the year 2000, there will be some 41 million people age 60 and over, comprising 15.5 percent of the total United States

---

[48]Nahemow and Lawton, "Toward an Ecological Theory of Adaptation and Aging," p. 319.

population, while those 65 years old and over will range somewhere between 11 percent and 13 percent of the population.[49]

We might note that increases in the old-age population are primarily the result of improvements in child care and disease prevention in early life. More people are surviving their infancy and thus reaching adulthood. Nevertheless, although more people are living longer, the expected increases in longevity, although substantial, are not spectacular.[50] It seems that life expectancy would be greatly increased only if certain medical breakthroughs were achieved. For example, it has been estimated that the elimination of death caused by cancer or stroke for persons age 65 and over would increase their life expectancy by 1½ years and that elimination of death caused by heart diseases would add as much as 5 years. The greatest impact on longevity would come from the elimination of the major cardiovascular renal diseases. If this were achieved, it is anticipated that 10 years could be added to life expectancy at age 65.[51]

two older populations

Because more people are reaching adulthood and because the death rate is gradually decreasing, we will soon have two groups of old people: the young–old and the old–old. For example, between 1940 and 1970 there was a 9 percent decrease in the proportion of the older population aged 65 through 74 years, whereas in the same period the relative number of those 75 through 84 years of age increased from 25 percent to over 30 percent. In addition, the 85-year-old-and-over portion of the population jumped from close to 4 percent of the aged in 1940 to 8 percent in 1970, accounting for some 1.5 million people.[52]

Thus, the older population is itself aging. This redistribution of age groups may greatly affect our concepts of "normal" life stages. For example, it suggests that we may begin to view the postretirement years as a *transition* stage into old age, which, in turn, may carry implications for discovering new developmental tasks through leisure.[53]

---

[49]U.S. Department of Health, Education, and Welfare, Statistical Memo No. 31, Publication (OHD) 75-20013, Washington, D. C., May, 1975.

[50]Ibid.

[51]H. B. Brotman, "Who Are the Aging?," in *Mental Illness in Later Life,* eds, E. W. Busse and E. Pfeiffer (Washington, D.C.: American Psychiatric Association, 1973).

[52]Ibid.

[53]Brok, "Issues in Leisure Relevant to Counseling and Applied Human Development."

distribution
of the older population by sex

It seems clear that the ratio of older women to older men has changed radically since the turn of the century. Table 3.3 gives the number of females per every 100 males 60 years old and over in the United States for the years 1900 and 1974.

Table 3.3   Number of females per 100 males 60 years and over in the United States in 1900 and 1974*

	Females per 100 Males	
Age	1900	1974
Total	97.0	133.8
60–64 years	95.3	114.1
65–74 years	95.7	130.1
75–84 years	101.0	160.9
85 years and over	125.4	202.1

*Adapted from U.S. Department of Health, Education, and Welfare, Statistical Memo No. 31, Publication (OHD) 75-20013, Washington, D.C., May, 1975 (Table B, p. 3).

Table 3.3 shows that the number of females per 100 males has increased dramatically since 1900. This trend is expected to continue through the year 2000. It is of interest that the greatest discrepancy between females and males appears in the older age categories. Thus, at age 85 and over there were (in 1974) more than two females for every male. It is anticipated that by the year 2000 this ratio will also hold for the 75-year-old-and-over category. Such trends obviously carry implications for female role definition, marital status, housing, and income policies.

income, education,
and living arrangements

Since there are some 22 million individuals over age 65 in the United States, the task of describing who the aged are might be easily subject to overgeneralizations. Twenty-two million people are not, and cannot, be all alike. In fact, it appears that as we grow older, individual differences are more likely to emerge.[54]

---

[54]Brotman, "Who Are the Aging?"

However, by looking at such factors as income levels, educational levels, and living arrangements in the aged, we may better realize that the elderly are somewhat alike. These factors remind us that the elderly, as a group, do, in fact, experience a different quality of life from their younger counterparts.

In terms of living arrangements, one fact stands out as obvious: The aged do not all live in nursing homes or institutions. Recent statistics indicate that only 5 percent of people over age 65 are institutionalized and that a large percentage of the noninstitutionalized aged are very active. Moreover, less than 1 percent of persons over age 65 are patients in mental hospitals and current estimates indicate that less than 10 percent of those living in and outside institutions have severe mental illness. Thus, the vast majority of those classified as older are not particularly hindered by unusual forms of mental illness. Additional information on living arrangements indicates that older women, compared to men, are more likely to live alone, due to the earlier death of their spouses.[55]

Older people have traditionally had less formal education than their younger counterparts. Recent estimates show that on average old people have had more than 4 years less schooling than younger members of the population (aged 25–64).[56] This trend is rapidly changing, however, and in the near future it is likely that old people will have as much (if not more as a result of the rise in continuing education) formal education as our nation's youth.

In terms of income, the aged comprise one of the poorest segments of our population. Recent statistics show that those who are 65 and over made up 14.6 percent of all the poor in the United States, while 16.3 percent of all old people are poor compared to 11.1 percent of people of all ages in the population. We must recall that poverty here is defined by the poverty threshold that is based on government standards and tied to the consumer price index. Recently this threshold was defined as an income of $2130 a year for a single person and $2680 a year for a couple. In fact, it has been estimated that more than one-half of the elderly suffer significant economic deprivation.[57]

---

[55]Gottesman, Quarterman, and Cohn, "Psychosocial Treatment of the Aged"; E. Palmore, "Social Factors in Mental Illness of the Aged," in *Mental Illness in Later Life*, eds., Busse and Pfeiffer; Brotman, "Who Are the Aging?"

[56]Brotman, "Who Are the Aging?"

[57]U.S. Department of Health, Education, and Welfare, *Facts and Figures on Older Americans*, No. 11, Publication (OHD) 75-20012, Washington, D.C., February 1975; S. Hume, *Basic Course in Gerontology* (Albany, N.Y.: School of Social Welfare, State University of New York at Albany, 1975).

The problems associated with income among the elderly have entered into the realm of treatment modalities. To some, for example, the most powerful intervention society can make in order to help the aged is to provide economic support. The importance of income is further reflected in the findings of a national sample of retirees that revealed that the most significant determination of postretirement satisfaction was having an adequate income.[58]

---

[58]Gottesman, Quarterman, and Cohn, "Psychosocial Treatment of the Aged"; R. Barfield and J. Morgan, *Early Retirement* (Ann Arbor, Mich.: Survey Research Center, 1968).

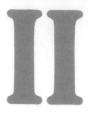

the
institutionalized
aged

4

the institutionalized aged

A recent report showed that there were 814,000 persons over 65 in institutions, only about 5 percent of all older people. Approximately one in seven was in a psychiatric facility; almost all of the rest were in nursing homes.[1] Studies have shown that the person who does enter the institution in later life is generally one who has been *chronically marginal,* i.e., he has not been able to cope adequately with the outside world in terms of utilizing existing support systems, such as family. These marginal people are alone and isolated. Although these people constitute but a small segment of today's elderly, it is on them that the commonly held stereotypes about aging are based. It is these stereotypes that make aging itself increasingly harder to accept as a normative process. In fact, there are those who regard aging as a disability. In this section we shall focus on that 5 percent of the institutionalized minority for whom aging *is* somewhat of a disability.

Institutionalization

Nursing homes like mental hospitals—or prisons—are *total institutions,* that, is "places of residence where a large number of like-situated individuals together lead an enclosed, formally administered round of life."[2] When one enters an institution, his

[1]L. E. Gottesman, C. E. Quarterman, and G. M. Cohn, "Psychosocial Treatment of the Aged," in *The Psychology of Adult Development and Aging,* eds., C. Eisdorfer and M. Lawton (Washington, D.C.: American Psychological Association, 1973).

[2]E. Goffman, *Asylums* (New York: Anchor Books, 1961), p. 1.

mastery or command over his world is disrupted; so much so that Goffman calls those who are institutionalized "inmates."

There occurs what Goffman terms a *mortification of self* in the form of the loss of roles, the loss of personal property, or even the loss of one's full name. There may be a disidentifying process, e.g., "I don't really belong here." This disidentification may be a reaction against "contaminative exposure," i.e., exposure to others who are less competent. In the nursing home one would anticipate this reaction from an alert resident who is exposed to a confused, regressed resident. One would also expect this as a reaction to the commonly held stereotype of the nursing home as a place to wait for death. These may partially explain why residents may be so detached from one another.

Moreover, in every institution there occurs a *looping process,* i.e., everything is fed back into everything else. Dress and manners, for example, are under constant scrutiny as are staff conversations and residents' conversations. The result is maximum visibility and minimum privacy. In addition, there exists in every institution a "caste system," i.e., an authoritarian staff class constantly doling out discipline to the residents. In reality, institutions are generally run according to staff convenience.

The sociological consequences of institutionalization have been aptly described.[3] It is no wonder that prolonged institutionalization is said to cause *desocialization.* Psychologically, an *institutional neurosis* has been described as a syndrome characterized by apathy, lack of initiative, lack of expression of feelings of resentment, lack of interest in the future, and deterioration of personal habits.[4] Thus, it is not surprising that many an institutionalized person is starved for some form of meaningful interaction that would improve the quality of his life.

who is the nursing home patient?

The median age of nursing home patients is 79.1 years. Seventy percent of nursing home patients are women, partially because they live longer than men and partially because women are more likely to remain widowed and alone. From 60 percent to 80 percent are poor, even though they may not have been poor before they were old. The vast majority have more than one chronic

---

[3]Ibid.

[4]J. Zusman, "Some Explanations of the Changing Appearance of Psychotic Patients," *International Journal of Psychiatry* **4** (1967): 216–237.

physical ailment. Nineteen percent have severe hearing defects and approximately 12 percent have severe visual impairments. Only one-sixth of all nursing home patients are confined to bed. It is estimated that one-half of those elderly who are confined to nursing homes have mental disorders or senility.[5]

chronic brain syndrome
and the institutionalized aging

The layman calls it *senility*. The professional calls it *chronic brain syndrome, organic brain syndrome, senile dementia,* or *senile psychosis*. All of these terms are likely to be applied to a large percentage of aging patients in long-term care facilities. These patients suffer various physical, cognitive, and emotional impairments and they exhibit symptoms of deterioration such as confusion, disorientation, faulty recent memory, emotional lability, indifference, poor interpersonal relationships, and apathy.

Despite various physical and physiological investigations and therapeutic attempts, the etiology of the symptoms (other than age) still remains unclear; however, the contributions of sensory impairment and social isolation have been recognized.[6] Monotony, boredom, and isolation often create similar symptoms in younger subjects; in older subjects these same conditions tend to heighten the symptoms of organic deterioration.[7]

No longer is there generalized espousal of the attitude that nothing can be done for the aging institutionalized person, for progress has been made in the alleviation of some of the symptoms of senility. Physical interventions have been tried, possibly with limited success but with success nonetheless. Trials have included anticoagulation therapy, hyperoxygenation, and vitamin B-12 administration.

In the affective domain, it has been demonstrated that even in very deteriorated, very old patients, intensified sensory input produced significant behavioral changes.[8] It is currently being recognized that senile signs may sometimes be behavioral manifestations of maladjustment, neuroticism, anxiety, and lack of

---

[5]R. Butler, *Why Survive? Being Old in America* (New York: Harper & Row, 1975); A.D. Haggarty, "The Role of the Long-Term Care Facility," in *A Practical Guide to Long-Term Care and Health Services Administration,* ed., M. Mitchel (Greenvale, N.Y.: Panel Publishers, 1973).

[6]D. A. Alexander, "Senile Dementia: A Changing Perspective," *British Journal of Psychiatry* **121** (1972): 207–214.

[7]C. A. Loew and B. M. Silverstone, "A Program of Intensified Stimulation and Response Facilitations for the Senile Aged," *The Gerontologist* **11** (1971): 341–347.

[8]Ibid.

ego strength resulting from a decline of participation in the environment and induced sensory deprivation. In fact, certain memory losses have been found to be selective. It has been suggested that some senile signs are, therefore, reversible.[9] However, if there is no appropriate intervention, senility becomes a vicious spiral, as shown in Fig. 4.1.

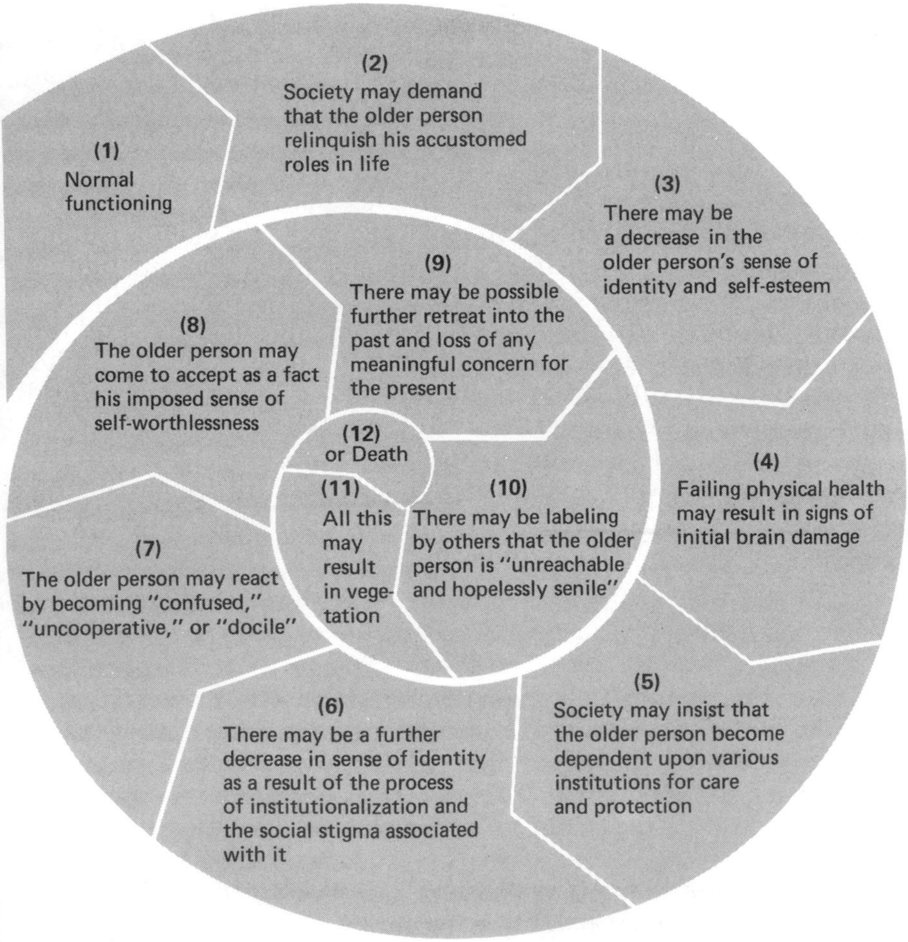

Figure 4.1 The spiral of senility. The patient may not go through all the stages shown nor in the order shown; however, all stages have been observed clinically in different patients at different times. Note that a consistently observed pattern in the spiral is the progressive decrease in self-esteem, ending in death. (*From* E. K. Barnes, A. Sack, and H. Shore, "Guidelines to Treatment Approaches," *Gerontologist* **13** (1973): 513–527)

---

[9]M. Oberleder, "Crisis Therapy in Mental Breakdown of the Aging," *The Gerontologist* **10** (1970): 111–114.

self-esteem

The sense of self that one develops in early life becomes a basic part of one's later personality and means of adapting to one's environment. Self-esteem builds from one's own achievements, activities, and sense of mastery. This sense of self is an important factor in determining the degree to which rejection, failure, physical illness, and stress can be tolerated. With aging and the accompanying stresses such as role loss, physical illness, financial insecurity, etc., there is decreased opportunity for the continued sense of mastery that is an essential ingredient of self-esteem.

This may be particularly true for the institutionalized aging person because the institutional complex may not lend itself to activities or personal interaction that build and help maintain one's self-esteem. In addition, choices within our institutions are limited so that one is given less opportunity to exercise a sense of self. Mastery of the environment is often not encouraged. Instead the institution pushes for the person to be the "good" patient, i.e., the patient who will show little incentive or little or no initiative and who will make little trouble for staff. It has been observed that this "model patient" often suffers from a decreased sense of worth. It is, therefore, no wonder that depression, with its accompanying feelings of worthlessness, is the most prevalent psychological problem found in older people.

depression

Depression may vary from feeling low to withdrawal or even suicide. Older people experiencing depression often state that during such times they feel discouraged, worried, or disgusted with their own uselessness. Often there are statements such as; "There is just no reason to go on living" or "I would welcome death."

Depression may often be masked and go unnoticed in the institutionalized older patient. This masking may be expressed by the patient's verbal listing of a host of somatic complaints. This is due, in part, to the fact that aging persons in our society are "allowed" to be sick and are often reinforced for this by the attention they receive from staff and others. Depressed persons may then have a host of people "fussing" over them only as long as they verbalize feelings of being ill. Since they state that they are depressed, others may move away from them without tuning into

[7]I. B. Lamm and J. C. Folsom, "Attitude Therapy and the Team Approach," *Mental Hospitals* **16** (1965): 307–320.

[8]Ibid., p. 311.

what could be behind the depression, such as feelings of anger turned inward or, most common, a type of mourning related to loss. Losses and declines are common in old age. The older person has less physical vitality, decreased mental agility, and decreased overall stamina. Of great impact are losses of other loved persons. These losses contribute greatly to feelings of social isolation and loneliness. These feelings of loneliness are often heightened when these people move into the impersonal institution. Along with this may also come distortions in body image.

body image

Closely related to the lack of self-esteem and feelings of depression are distortions of body image. These relate to misconceptions of one's sexual identity, one's size, one's strength, and one's beauty, e.g., "I am too short for anyone to love me," "I am ugly," "I am weak." These distortions or devaluations are not a function of aging per se, but rather a compilation of earlier experiences, e.g., past successes or failures, good or bad health, affection or neglect, love or dislike.

In a series of studies concerned with measuring the body image of six groups, four geriatric and two younger groups, with an overall age range of from 18 to 90 years, it was found that one of the oldest groups, with a mean age of 83 and residing in a home for the aged, scored lowest on indices measuring body worries and body discomforts whereas a younger group residing in a mental hospital scored the highest.[10] In a study of body image as related to assigned dollar values for hypothetically lost body parts, it was found that there was no significant relationship between age and the dollar value placed on either individual parts or the average for all body parts. Again, psychiatric patients placed significantly less value on their bodies than did persons who did not have psychiatric disorders, regardless of age. Together, these findings imply that by itself advanced age plays a less prominent role in impaired body image than do psychiatric status and environmental factors such as lack of stimulation. Further studies also tend to support this implication.[11]

---

[10]R. Plutchik, M. B. Weiner, and H. Conte, "Studies of Body Image I: Body Worries and Body Discomforts," *Journal of Gerontology* **26** (1971): 344–350.

[11]R. Plutchik, H. Conte, and M. B. Weiner, "Studies of Body Image II: Dollar Values of Body Parts, *Journal of Gerontology* **28** (1973): 89–91; R. Plutchik, H. Conte, and M. B. Weiner, "Studies of Body Image III: Body Feelings as Measured by the Semantic Differential," *International Journal of Aging and Human Development* **4** (1973): 378–380.

sensory deprivation

We are becoming more and more aware that people require
not only stimulation but also varied sensory input for the
maintenance of normal, adaptive behavior, Initial experiments
attesting to this were conducted at McGill University in 1953.
McGill students were paid $20 a day to remain in an environment
that induced sensory deprivation. Despite the high rate of pay,
subjects could not remain in that environment more than two to
three days. During the experiment much restlessness and
emotional liability were observed and after the experiment was
over students reported that they had had disturbances in visual,
auditory, and perceptual spheres and hallucinations during the
experiment. These data seemed to provide direct evidence for an
intense dependence on one's environment that had not been
previously recognized. Once a person is placed in an environment
that lacks stimulation a form of psychological suspended animation
appears to take place.[12]

In linking sensory deprivation experiments to aging, a study
was performed in Australia involving sensory stimulation for the
treatment of what is termed *senile dementia*. Results of this study
seem to confirm the fact that senile dementia may be only partially
influenced by actual pathological changes occurring in the brain; it
may be largely influenced by sensory deprivation that accompanies
the disease. In addition, this deprivation may in large measure be
the result of decreased social interaction. The authors suggest that
stimulation in the environment may either slow down or, at times,
reverse this process. Thus, lack of stimulation may be another
contributing factor to chronic brain syndrome, perhaps one that
could possibly be reduced by various intervention strategies.[13]

[12]W. H. Bexton, W. Heron, and T. H. Scott, "Effects of Decreased Variation in the
Sensory Environment," *Canadian Journal of Psychology* 8 (1954): 70–76.

[13]H. M. Bower, "Sensory Deprivation with Aged: Sensory Stimulation and the
Treatment of Senile Dementia," *Exerpta Medica-Gerontology and Geriatrics* 2 (1968): 352.

5

rehabilitation: the step-ladder approach

Intervention Strategies

There are many psychosocial rehabilitative strategies, e.g., activities therapy, music therapy, drama therapy, poetry therapy, body movement therapy, and art thereapy—so many that it is almost like alphabet soup! Persons who have a wide range of skills and a wide range of educational and experiential backgrounds use various techniques. However, despite their diversity, all techniques share certain characteristics: (1) psychosocial stimulation; (2) opportunities for social interaction; and (3) opportunities for positive reinforcement related to growth and achievements, all of which are necessary ingredients of comprehensive care and which may mitigate against the negative effects of institutionalization.

All of the therapies mentioned above, though not a complete list, may be appropriate to patients who are considered to be fairly intact. (These therapies will be discussed later.) They are generally led by fairly specialized personnel. In addition, they may also be used in conjunction with each other and along with a wide variety of modalities, as shown in Fig. 5.1.

The techniques we shall focus on here, and in the chapters to follow, Sensory Training, Reality Orientation, and Remotivation, are geared especially toward the more regressed, less intact patient. It may be recalled that one-half of all nursing home patients have some form of mental disorder or senility. The techniques are also to be used sequentially so that when each one is successfully completed, it leads to the next one. We have labeled this approach the *step-ladder approach*.

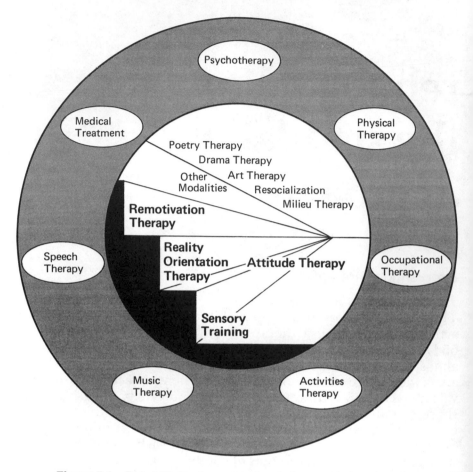

Figure 5.1   Rehabilitation is a many-faceted concept wherein various interventions may be used simultaneously.

the step-ladder approach
to rehabilitation

The step-ladder approach can be used to match treatment modalities to the various levels of patient functioning. In the step-ladder approach a very regressed patient is assigned to a basic treatment technique and then is moved up the ladder, that is, assigned to successively more complex techniques once he has experienced success on these lower levels.

Since chronic brain syndrome patients may be on a progressively downhill course, success may be minimal. In fact, there may be regression. In general, however, it has been clinically observed that patients are able to progress from one step to another.

Before looking at each technique in detail, a brief description of each follows.

Sensory training. Sensory training is a structured group/individual experience that involves all five senses, a technique that is used with the regressed older person who shows an inability to interact with his environment. The goal is to bring this individual back in touch with his surroundings by providing varied stimuli to improve the patient's response to his environment.

Reality orientation. Reality orientation is a structured common-sense behavioral approach to rehabilitating acutely or moderately confused patients to their immediate surroundings. The goal is to help them relearn basic information about themselves and their environment in order to improve their general orientation, i.e., awareness of time, place and person.

Remotivation therapy. Remotivation therapy is a structured program of group discussion that encourages individuals to take renewed interest in their surroundings by focusing their attention on the simple, objective features of everyday life by means of a single relearning process.

These three techniques are a basic core of programs for patients who are less intact than others and who are unable to benefit sufficiently from the full range of program offerings. As a result of the participation in these specialized, highly structured group programs, it is hoped that social interaction skills will be improved and that increased participation in other activities will become possible.

Matching Patients to Treatments:
A "Best Fit" Concept

We can now be concerned with understanding which kind of patient is best suited to which technique. This insures that the technique most suited to an individual patient at a given time will be the one assigned to him. Matching patients to a particular technique or therapy may be redone at several points in time.

the severely regressed patient:
the first step

Some patients appear to be more regressed because they are apathetic and withdrawn. This patient often spends most of his time in his room or seeming to be asleep in an upright position during the day and relatively inattentive to his surroundings. Staff may refer to this person as being "pretty much out of things." It may be that his behavior is a result of either organic processes or of an environment that is devoid of stimulation or a result of both factors. The end result, however, is that this patient appears to be relatively inactive and uninvolved.

If we take a developmental approach to the patient, we can see that this patient would benefit most from sensory input. For example, the infant requires a great deal of stroking, caressing, and cuddling early in life. Although the geriatric patient is not to be infantilized, at the same time he may require the same kinds of "stroking" as a result of his particular situation during these later years. Not having experienced much touching or interaction with others, he may now require this sensory input. The stroking and reinforcement for alertness are crucial to the patient.

When the patient is defined as being relatively regressed, he would be considered a likely candidate for the first technique in the step-ladder approach—sensory training. In order to determine if a patient best fits into this category, staff should confer with those who are most in contact with this patient in order to obtain a general evaluation. If there is a designated team leader, which is the case in many facilities, this team leader would assign the patient to the modality of sensory training.

the moderately regressed patient:
the second step

The patient appropriate for this technique is one who may have a good deal of difficulty in the cognitive sphere. He would tend to be confused and disoriented about time, place, and person. This may be the chronic brain syndrome patient, the poststroke patient, or the patient who has experienced head trauma. Using the developmental approach, we may assume that this level relates to the young child who has less need of the stroking and caressing gestures we spoke of earlier and is now being "talked to" by the parenting figure. Speech is used as a means of orienting the child to the world and familiarizing him in a total way with his environment.

Similarly, the geriatric patient has, because of both organic processes and environmental changes, been given less attention and may therefore have lost his former reality based orientation to the world. When the structure of the environment is not communicated often and in a continuous way, as is often the case in institutions, it may be that there is no need to know that "Monday" is "Monday" and that this is different from "Saturday." Our real world consists not only of abstract knowledge of the world but structures within each day that bring home the fact that, for example, Monday is a workday and that Sunday is part of a nonwork weekend. When the geriatric patient is in an environment in which one day leads into another and in which there are no boundaries or structures to define what it is that makes up that day, there may be a sense of loss of "day-ness," "time-ness," "place-ness," etc. It is this patient who is best suited for reality orientation therapy.

Again, as with the patient assigned to sensory training, the best way to determine if a patient is most suited for reality orientation is to talk to the patient. The worker can ask for simple information such as; What day is it today? What is the weather like? What holiday is coming? If the patient has difficulty in most of these areas, the worker can assume that the patient is suited to reality orientation therapy.

Sometimes it is difficult to determine if the patient should be assigned a lower level technique, such as sensory training, or a slightly higher one, such as reality orientation. It has been found that the best way to determine this is to assess which of the behaviors formerly mentioned are most characteristic of the patient. That is, does he seem so withdrawn that sensory awakening would be helpful to him or does he seem to have no problem in this area but have difficulties in orientation. Again, although the patient may show signs of needing both, it is best to assign him to that treatment modality that seems to be the one he needs the *most* at the particular time.

It has also been suggested that since these techniques are arranged hierarchically, i.e., sensory training is the lower level one with the other techniques ranked above it, it is best, when in doubt, to assign the patient a lower level technique at first. This step-ladder approach prevents insulting the patient's sense of himself. The patient would not be assigned a higher level technique and then be "demoted." That is, it is best that the patient be assigned a lower level technique with the possibility that the worker underestimated the patient's functional level and can then reassign him or promote him upward.

A reliable and valid scale for measuring the degree of overall functioning in geriatric patients is the *geriatric rating scale*.[1] This scale is easy to administer because it can be done on the wards by staff personnel and it requires no special training on the part of the rater. In addition, the patient need not be cooperative or even present during the rating (see Appendix A). This scale has been found helpful in ascertaining the characteristics of geriatric patients prior to their participation in such programs as sensory training and reality orientation therapy.

the least regressed patient:
the third step

Remotivation therapy follows reality orientation. Using our developmental model, we can think of the young child who is now in a classroom setting. Having been stroked and talked to by parenting figures, he is now in a structured environment in which he is learning about the real world. Similarly, the geriatric patient may be in need of a structured group setting in which his intellectual interest in the world is restimulated. Again, as with sensory training and reality orientation, the worker can best gain an understanding of the technique most suited to the patient by talking with the patient and other staff. The geriatric rating scale may also be helpful.

This form of therapy is a structured technique that includes definitive steps that must be followed. In many ways it is similar to a classroom experience with a teacher (the worker) and with students (the geriatric patients). In other words, the worker uses a prepared folder similar to a class lesson plan. The exercise also asks for concrete information of a "school" nature. The topics include stamps, holidays, travel, fashions, etc. Focus is on the accuracy of the response. In addition, whereas in sensory training therapy and reality orientation therapy individual attention is given each patient, here the focus, though individual, is on the group. The patients are not stroked and are not touched as in the preceding techniques. The patient to be chosen for this technique is one who is regarded as functioning on a higher level than the patients in either of the two preceding groups.

---

[1]R. Plutchik, H. Conte, M. Lieberman, M. B. Weiner, J. Grossman, and N. Lehrman, "Reliability and Validity of a Scale for Assessing the Functioning of Geriatric Patients," *Journal of the American Geriatrics Society* **18** (1970): 491–499.

6

sensory training

Background and Goals

Sensory training is used effectively with the regressed older person who shows an inability to interact with his environment. The goal is to literally bring this individual back in touch with his surroundings. Sensory training is a structured group/individual experience that involves all five senses. The aim is to provide the older person with differentiated stimuli to improve his perception of, and response to, both the physical and human environments. This technique, developed by Leona Richman in 1968 when she was Director of Occupational Therapy at Bronx Psychiatric Center, is geared to the more regressed geriatric patient who was formerly afforded little opportunity for activity or group participation with trained staff.

The more regressed patient residing in a rehabilitative setting had little or no treatment modalities available to him, but the better functioning patients were able to take advantage of such activities as occupational therapy, recreational therapy, activities of daily living, psychotherapy, and other modalities. These activities, however, required a long attention span, small and large muscle control, perceptual motor coordination, socialization skills, and the ability to follow instructions. Thus, only the more able, self-motivated patients could take advantage of the available rehabilitative activities.

Sensory training attempts to combat the effects of physical, social, and psychological breakdown in the more regressed geriatric patient by either maintaining the level the patient is at or by avoiding further decompensation. Sensory training breaks the

environment into its most simplified and comprehensible form.
Simple body awareness exercises and sensory stimuli are
presented, experienced, reacted to, and understood by the
patients. The environment then becomes predictable and
"deconfused." The peers with whom the patient is interacting,
along with the leader, provide an opportunity for interaction, for
recognition by others and, most essentially, for feedback on
behavior that may then be amenable to change.

The Target Population

Patients appropriate for this technique exhibit deficiencies in any
or all of the following areas: perceptual motor ability, sensory input
discrimination, and psychosocial performance. Thus, the
regressed patient who is socially withdrawn, for example, would
benefit from sensory training. Verbal proficiency is not necessary
and patients who lack the use of one of the senses, e.g., the blind or
the deaf, should not be excluded from the group because the
training experience will help them to learn to use the other senses
more efficiently and to compensate for the original loss.

Composition of the Group

Ideally, there should be between five and seven patients in a group
and there should be a balance of verbal and nonverbal members.
Nevertheless, a group may function well with as few as four
members or as many as ten.

Optimally, a group should consist of members who are at the
same level of functioning. In order to determine which patients are
best suited for this technique, there should be consultations with
the staff members who are most in contact with the patient on a
daily basis. It must be determined whether or not the patient is
having difficulty interacting with his environment mostly because
of his sensory loss. It is best when several staff members agree that a
particular patient would benefit most from sensory training at this
particular time.

Not all patients have to be at the same level of regression. It is
often helpful to have a "sparker" in the group, i.e., a member who
can, by his level of participation, enthusiasm, interest, and rapport
with the leader, help keep the group lively. He may also function as
a model for others to imitate.

Time

Experienced staff suggested that the best time for sensory training is in the morning because patients are generally well rested and are more alert. The day may be started with sensory awakening and awareness as a preparation for the rest of the day. The group session may last approximately an hour, although the initial sessions may be shorter because of the patients' short attention span and unfamiliarity with the group experience. Later, as the group becomes more cohesive and as the members become more comfortable with each other and with the experience, the session may last longer. Time of day, however, may have to be modified to best suit the needs of the patient, the staff, and the institutional schedules. For example, if the physical therapist comes only in the morning and if members of the group receive physical therapy, the morning would not be the appropriate time. If patients try to leave the group during the first few sessions because they get restless, it may be helpful to shorten the length of the session. A shorter session is better than no session at all, and shorter sessions at more frequent intervals are still better.

Frequency

The most progress may be seen if the session is conducted every day, seven days a week. If this is not feasible, five times a week is also very beneficial. In some facilities, however, there are as few as two sessions per week. The number of times per week, like the time afforded each session, will be determined as a function of the support of the administration, other duties of the leader, other activities offered to this patient group and, in general, the total schedule of the institution. Thus, total familiarity with the various institutional activities, e.g., meal times, bath times, religious services, visiting, is necessary in order for the leader to choose a time that does not conflict with other programs.

Place

The group should meet in the same place every time. The room used should be quiet, comfortable, and well lit. It should be somewhat out of the way so that the group is not distracted by other patients or staff. It should be a room that the group members can think of as *their* meeting place for sensory training. The room should not be too large or cluttered and the atmosphere should be one of intimacy. Chairs should be arranged in a circle to allow for the most interaction among members and to permit members to observe each other. This affords the most involvement in terms of a total sharing experience of both a verbal and nonverbal nature. The chairs should have enough room between them so that the group leader may feel free to move around between them but they should not be so distant that the closeness of the group situation is lost. Patients in wheelchairs should be included in the circle and there should be sufficient space between the wheelchairs so that the leader can move around between them.

Materials for Sensory Training

No special materials are needed for the exercises. Simple everyday objects are suggested for the sensory stimulation portion. For example, for the sense of smell one could bring in a freshly cut flower, some tobacco, or some perfume. To stimulate hearing, one could bounce a ball, clap hands, or ring a bell. For touch, one could use sandpaper, a piece of velvet, a piece of Brillo, or a piece of cotton. For vision, one could use a hand mirror or a set of different colored and/or shaped objects. For taste, the options are wide. One could reinforce the sessions by offering goodies or refreshments at the end of the session.

The major point here is that *nothing special* has to be *purchased.* One could use what is readily available in the facility. The primary factor is the leader's interest and creativity.

A Written Schedule or Reinforcement

It has been found most useful to have the schedule of the sensory training's time, day, and place and the names of the participants posted in conspicuous places on the ward. This tends to remind staff, patients, the administration, visitors, and all others that sensory training is being conducted or that "something is happening on the wards." It also helps patients to remember where they are to go, at what time, and on what day. It reinforces memory because it activates memory traces that could otherwise become stale through disuse.

It has been found most helpful to have these listings displayed in several places along the ward, such as near the day room, outside the nurses' quarters, and outside the area where the sensory training session is being held. The best way to exhibit these names, times, days, etc., is to write them in large block letters in dark ink to insure maximum visibility.

The Leader

The leader, or the one trained in the sensory training technique, may be a staff member, a volunteer, or even another patient. Sensory training sessions are conducted by people from a variety of disciplines such as nursing, occupational therapy, recreational therapy, physical therapy, social work, and psychology. Volunteers may also learn and apply this technique. In addition, it has been found that occasionally more intact patients can learn this approach and be used as ancillary therapists. In other words, any person who is motivated and believes that the regressed geriatric patient can be helped by therapeutic approaches may learn and apply this technique successfully. The leader of a particular group should remain with that group as consistently as possible. Since there may be several sensory training groups conducted throughout a given facility by a variety of staff, these leaders should exchange information and experiences regularly in order to better understand how their patients are progressing.

Role of the Leader During a Session

The leader is responsible for establishing a friendly, nonthreatening atmosphere. The group members should find each session a comfortable, positive, and rewarding experience. The leader accomplishes this by accepting patients as they are and by emphasizing their abilities and contributions through reinforcing the right responses and ignoring the incorrect responses. Eye contact is used as much as possible. The group leader may have to squat at the side of the patient he is working with in order to establish and maintain eye contact when speaking with him. The group leader who has a "warm" quality and who can easily touch his patients has been found to be successful with the patient who is going through sensory training.

It should be emphasized that sensory training is *not* primarily a classroom or teaching situation and that the correctness of the response is not the prime factor. What is important is the patient's experience within the context of the total group situation. Different members of the group may perceive the same stimulus in various ways. The leader is not to correct the participant because he gives the "wrong" answer. Instead, each member's perceptions are to be accepted and appreciated. In this way, the patient feels free to offer responses and gets reinforcement with each response. This encourages building self-confidence and self-esteem, essential components of the total group experience.

Sensory Training Technique

orientation

The first part of the sensory training technique consists of *orientation*. The leader greets each individual member by name and introduces each member to the rest of the group. Although first names usually help to establish an informal atmosphere, the leader should be sensitive to his patients' feelings about this and use surnames whenever he feels that a patient needs this kind of respect. It has sometimes been helpful for the leader to say something like, "Shall I call you Mrs. C. or Sara? Which do you prefer?" The leader must sensitively use his own judgment. Name tags are helpful for both patients and the leader. They should be written in large letters so that they can be read easily. Both the patient's first and second name should be on the tag.

The leader should comment on something each of the members is wearing or comment on the consistency of attendance at the meetings because these comments make each person feel welcome and they reinforce positive behavior. Remarks such as, "Mrs. G., you look so nice with your hair combed that way" or "Mr. S., it is so good to see you coming to all of these sessions" have proven helpful.

Once greetings have been concluded, the group is then oriented to the time and place. For example, the leader may say, "Today is Monday, June 5th and we are meeting in the day room of XYZ Place." The leader then tells the group the purpose of the meeting, i.e., that they are there to do exercises and that they will be doing two kinds of exercises, for the body and for the mind. The leader then outlines for the group the benefits of doing exercises and why it is important for everyone to do them. He may state,

"These exercises help us identify our body parts" or, "Our exercises for our mind help us remember and that makes us feel good." Having thus been introduced and oriented to the time, place, and purpose, the group is ready to begin exercising.

body awareness exercises

The second segment of the session consists of the body awareness exercises. During this portion of the session the different body joints are identified. The leader may say, "We are now going to exercise our wrists. Here is my wrist and this is how it moves." The major purpose of this is to give the patients a sense of body awareness and explain to them the obvious benefits of moving body parts that might ordinarily remain motionless. It has been found that it is more important for the group members to be able to identify their body parts than to do the actual exercises. Whenever possible, each member of the group should do the exercise.

Specifically, the joints on the arm to be exercised are the shoulders, elbows, wrists, and fingers. The legs are exercised by moving the knees and the ankles. The neck and the waist might also be exercised. It is important for the leader to follow a structured sequence when he introduces each joint. He should progress from the top of the body (shoulders) to the bottom (ankles). There is then a review in which the leader verbalizes what has just been done, e.g., "We have just finished exercising our wrists."

stimulation of the senses

The third segment involves *sensory stimulation*. In this phase the five senses and their corresponding sensory organs are identified. These senses are stimulated by a variety of props (a flower, a cookie, a mirror brought in by the leader or found in the room) and are reacted to by the group members. It is essential that each sense be stimulated in each session and that each group member has an opportunity to respond to each stimulus.

The leader should start with sight and end with taste. The group members are told that they will exercise the sense of sight, for example, by using their eyes. The leader identifies his own eyes and helps the group members find theirs. The group may then be presented with something to see (a mirror) and asked to respond to, not identify, what they see. Questions such as "Do you like what you see?" or "How do you look today?" may be asked. The leader then repeats to the entire group what the individual group member said, such as, "Sara said she looks nice today" or "Mr. J. says he sees his own face." Not only does this stimulate sight, but it also heightens self-awareness.

Taste may be left for last since the stimulus serves as a reward, e.g., a sucking candy or cookie for those whose diets permit this (other foods are used for those whose diets do not permit sweets). Group members usually enjoy this very much.

The leader encourages appropriate responses by phrasing questions that are in accord with each individual's level of functioning. Thus, better functioning patients may be able to answer a question such as, "How does this smell?" when presented with the odor of tobacco or perfume. This question might be difficult for a lower functioning patient to answer. The leader might ask this patient, "Can you smell this?" or "Do you like this smell?" These questions require little cognitive ability, i.e., the simple identification of the odor, and allow a nonverbal patient the opportunity to respond. When the patient does respond to a presented stimulus, e.g., the sound of the ball being bounced by the leader, the leader repeats the patient's verbal response to the entire group. When the response is nonverbal (a shaking of the head indicating "yes" to the question "Do you like this smell?"), this response is also interpreted for all to share. The leader may shake his head and say, "Sara is shaking her head because she likes this smell."

conclusion

The final segment of the session is termed the conclusion. Here the leader asks the group for feedback on their enjoyment of the session. He may repeat some of the members' comments. Before he concludes the session the leader announces the time and place for the next meeting and thanks each member for coming. He may use a personal greeting for each group member along with general comments, such as, "Thank you for coming. I hope that you enjoyed it. See you next (day) at (time) o'clock at (place)."

Immediately after the conclusion of the entire session the group leader should complete a written evaluation of what has happened while it is still fresh in his mind (see Appendix B). It is most essential that the evaluation be made *before* the leader's memory fades. It also insures there being a written documentation of progress over time. The documentation makes it easier for staff to understand how the group experience has affected the level of functioning of a particular patient. It is direct evidence of a line of growth that has to be charted in order to be fully understood. It also serves as a record to be used for determining if the patient should continue in this technique, or, perhaps, be promoted to the next one. Record keeping is most essential whether the leader uses the evaluation forms provided or makes up his own.

Primary and Secondary Levels of Sensory Training

There are two levels of sensory training: primary and secondary. The primary level is used for the more regressed and withdrawn patients. It is concrete and extremely structured and the tasks are simple. The leader, using this level, tells the group members everything instead of asking them questions. There is one simple exercise for each body part, usually involving an "in–out" or an "up–down" motion and there is one concrete stimulus for each sense. The leader uses a stimulus that the participants find easy to respond to, for example, a loud noise (the banging of a hammer), a harsh smell (ammonia), or a rough texture (a brush). The patients at this level are asked only if they can experience the stimulus ("Can you smell this?") and if they like what they are experiencing ("Do you like the smell?").

At the second level, called secondary sensory training, the leader adheres to the same basic structure as that outlined above but here he makes the tasks more challenging. He tells the group less and he asks more in order to encourage more participation because these group members are more able to participate. Thus, he might ask, "Why is it important for us to do these exercises?" In addition, he might introduce two exercises for each body part or even ask group members to suggest some exercises to do. He might present two sensory stimuli for each sense and ask the patient to compare the two. Wording, too, may be different. For example, the leader may introduce an adjective into the question by asking the group member to choose the adjective he prefers. For example, "Does it smell weak or strong?" "Does it feel rough or smooth?" As suggested previously, the leader repeats the group member's answer so that all members of the group will be aware of the particular response.

primary sensory training session

The following is an example of how a leader might conduct a primary sensory training session.

Leader:	Good morning everyone. Today we are going to do some exercises. But first, let us introduce ourselves. My name is ———.

> [*To first group member.*]

Would you please tell us your name.

> [*Leader stands just to the side of the patient so that others can see.*]

Patient:	My name is Joseph.
Leader:	This is Joseph. I am glad that you could join us today, Joseph.

> [*To next group member.*]

Would you like to tell us your name, please.

Leader: I said that today we are here to do exercises. We are going to do two kinds of exercises, exercises for our bodies and exercises for our minds. First we will exercise our bodies and then we will exercise our minds. Exercising makes us feel healthy and keeps us limber. We are going to exercise the parts of the body that move called the joints. The first part that we will exercise is the shoulders.

> [*Touches shoulders.*]

These are my shoulders. Can you find your shoulders? Joseph, these are your shoulders.

> [*Touches Joseph's shoulders.*]

Good, Mary is now showing us where her shoulders are. John has found his shoulders. Betty, here are your shoulders.

> [*Touches Betty's shoulders.*]

Now that we have all found our shoulders, we will exercise them. We will exercise our shoulders by moving our arms up and down.

> [*Raises arms up over head and then lowers them down to side. Moves around the circle, helping those having difficulty and offering both verbal and tactile or touch praise.*]

Good. Now that we have exercised our shoulders, we will exercise our elbows. These are my elbows. Can you find your elbows?

[Repeats as with shoulders.]

This process is repeated and similar wording is used for all the joints from the shoulders down to the ankles. Modifications may be used by the group leader, depending on his awareness of the needs of his particular group.

Leader: We have just finished exercising our ankles and that completes our body exercises. We exercised our shoulders, elbows, wrists, fingers, knees, and ankles.

[As the leader reviews these joints, he moves around the circle, touching one member's shoulder, another's elbow, etc., for demonstration purposes.]

How do you feel after having done these exercises?

[Typical responses are "tired," "O.K.," "good," etc.]

Now we are going to exercise our minds. It is important to exercise our minds because we think with our minds and our minds tell us a lot about the world around us. We will exercise our minds by using our five senses. The five senses are seeing—with our eyes; hearing—with our ears; smelling—with our noses; touching—with our fingers; and tasting—with our tongues.

[Again, as the leader lists the sensory organs, he moves around the circle, touching one person's eyes, another's nose, etc.]

The first sense that we will use is seeing and we see with our eyes.

[Points to his own eyes.]

Can everyone find their eyes?

[Leader helps those who have difficulty finding their eyes and offers praise for all as they point to their eyes.]

Now I have something here that we are going to see with our eyes. This is a mirror and we use a mirror to see ourselves. Joseph, I'd like you to look in the mirror, please. Can you see yourself?

[Leader kneels to the side of the patient and holds the mirror so that Joseph can see his reflection if Joseph cannot hold the mirror himself. If the patient can hold the mirror himself, he is encouraged to do so.]

How do you look today?

[Leader repeats the response to the group.]

Mary, can you see yourself in the mirror?

[Each patient then gets an opportunity to look in the mirror and to respond to this stimulus.]

Now that we have used our eyes to see, we are going to use our noses to smell. This is my nose. Where is your nose?

[Again the leader helps those who have difficulty locating their noses and offers both tactile and verbal praise to all.]

I have something here I'd like you to smell. Tell me if you like it.

[Leader holds stimulus so that everyone can see it and so that no one is taken by surprise.]

Mary, I have something here for you to smell. Can you smell it?

[Waits for response.]

Do you like the smell?

[Both the response to this and the preceding question are repeated to the group. Each member gets a chance to respond to the stimulus. Responses are always repeated for the group.]

So far we have exercised our eyes to see and our noses to smell. Now we will use our ears to hear.

[Members are asked to locate this sensory organ.]

I have a mallet and I am going to make a noise with it.

[Leader bangs once sharply.]

Did everyone hear that? Now I am going to make that noise a number of times and I'd like everyone to listen with their ears and try to count the number of times you hear it.

[Leader bangs from two to five times distinctly and asks each member how many times he heard the noise. If one patient says that he heard a different number of bangings from another patient, the difference is not noted. What is important is that each patient did hear the noise.]

We have exercised our sense of seeing, smelling, and hearing. Now we will exercise our sense of touch by using our fingers. These are my fingers. Show me yours. I have a brush. I am going to rub you across your fingers with this brush.

[Holding the brush so that all can see.]

I would like you to tell me if you like the way that the brush feels. Joseph, I am going to rub you with the brush.
[Holds the patient's hand palm facing up and rubs the patient's fingers with the brush lightly.]
Can you feel this? Do you like the way it feels?
[Repeat response to the group.]
The last sense that we will exercise is the sense of taste. To taste we use our tongues. This is my tongue. Where is yours? I have something that I would like you all to taste.
[Leader passes out stimulus to all patients and then asks for individual responses.]
Mary, can you taste the candy? How does it taste to you?
[Responses are repeated for the group.]
Well, today we have done a lot of exercises. We exercised our bodies and we exercised our minds by using our five senses. Did you enjoy doing these exercises? Shall we do them again? We will do them again tomorrow morning at ten o'clock. Thank you all for coming.
[Leader shakes each member's hand, thanks each one for coming, and makes an appropriate and rewarding personal comment to each member of the group.]

secondary
sensory training session

The following is an example of how a leader might conduct a secondary sensory training session.

Leader: Good morning everyone. Today we are going to do some exercises. But first let us introduce ourselves. Does anyone remember my name?
[Stands behind a patient's chair.]
Now, does anyone remember this lady's name?
[Stands behind another patient's chair.]
Now, what is this man's name? Good.
[Leader says "good" if the patient is correct; if the patient is wrong, he does not allude to the mistake but goes on to ask another patient. If this too proves unsuccessful, the leader may state the person's name himself.]
Does anyone know what today's date is?
[Uses technique as above until he gets the correct response from a

group member; if this does not happen within a reasonable time, the leader gives the correct answer himself.]
What is the name of this place that we are all in?
[*Again uses the technique described for giving person's name and date.*]
We are going to do two kinds of exercises today. First, we will exercise our bodies and then we will exercise our minds. Is it important to exercise our bodies? Why is it so important?
[*Gets a response from one of the members.*]
Good. We will exercise the parts of our bodies that move called the joints. Can anyone remember the first part of our body that we exercised? Good. Yes, it is the shoulders. Can anyone show us how we exercise the shoulders?
[*Waits for response.*]
Good.
Now that we have exercised our bodies, we will exercise our minds. Why is it important to exercise our minds?
[*Waits for appropriate response from a group member.*]
Good. We will exercise our minds by using the five senses. Does anyone remember any of the five senses?
[*Waits for response and reinforces an appropriate one.*]
The first sense that we will exercise is the sense of seeing. What do we use to help us see? We use our eyes. John, how many people do you see in this room? Is anyone wearing red clothing? Is anyone in this room wearing blue clothing?
[*Again reinforces appropriate response.*]
Can anyone see anything in the room that has a square shape? A round shape?

Other examples of vision exercises that may be used are (1) Simon Says; (2) describing the appearance of others in the group and their clothing; (3) describing the colors, furnishings, and decorations (such as paintings) in the room.

Leader: Now we will exercise the sense of hearing. What do we use to hear with? Am I speaking in a loud voice or in a soft voice? Mary, say "hello" to Pat in a loud voice. Now Pat, say "hello" to Mary in a soft voice.
[*Technique continues as before, with repeating of response and reinforcement of it.*]

I'd like everyone to close their eyes and try to identify the noise that I make.

[*Noises to be made may be in the form of keys rattling, paper crumpling, door slamming, hands clapping, or whistling.*]

I'd like everyone to close their eyes. I am going to make a loud noise and I would like everyone to listen and tell me from which part of the room the noise is coming.

Now we will exercise our sense of smell. What do we use to smell with? What are some of the things that smell good to you? What are some of the things that smell bad to you?

I have two things here that I would like you to smell.

[*Has perfume and turpentine.*]

Which smell do you like better? Which is stronger? Can you identify them?

The next sense that we will exercise is the sense of touching. What do we use to touch with? John, can you touch Mary's hands? Do they feel warm or cold? Mary, how do John's hands feel?

[*Holds Mary's hand.*]

Whose hand is warmer, John's or mine?

I have two objects here that I would like you to feel.

[*Rubs patient with sandpaper and silk.*]

Roberta, which is smoother?

I have a bag here filled with different objects (pencil, ball, cup, toothbrush, safety pin, button). I'd like you to reach into the bag, grab an object, and with your eyes closed try to identify the object just by touching it.

[*As always, appropriate responses are reinforced and repeated to the group.*]

The last sense that we will exercise today is the sense of taste. What do we use to taste with? I have two things here (cracker and a sourball candy) that I would like you to taste.

[*Hands each one a cracker.*]

What kind of a taste does that have?

[*Hands each one a sourball after making sure that this and the cracker are allowed on everyone's diet.*]

What kind of taste does that have? Which taste did you like better?

[*In addition, the leader might have the patients identify different flavors in a pack of Life Saver candies.*]

Those are the exercises for today. How did you enjoy
these exercises? Shall we do them again? We will do them
again tomorrow morning at ten o'clock. Thank you all
for coming.

[*Shakes each patient's hand as he leaves and again offers each
one a personal statement.*]

Innovations in Technique:
Using Associations

It has been found helpful to use associations in secondary level
sensory training sessions. For example, after he has been stroked
with a brush, a patient may be asked, "What does it remind you of?"
Similarly, after being stroked with velvet, a patient might say that it
feels "soft" or "cuddly." A patient who has been encouraged to
associate might say, "Like a dress I used to have. I wore it at a
wedding a long time ago." The leader may then go on to stimulate
other memories such as when the wedding took place, whose
wedding it was, the color of the dress, the meaning of the event to
the patient. This modification allows the patient to reminisce, thus
providing additional meaning to the sensory training experience
and reactivating the memory traces of her former life, linking past
and present. In all, association adds an additional integrative
function for the patient.

The leader should use associations to heighten the experience
of each group member, trying to give one an opportunity to
associate and reinforcing each with comments like, "It sounds like
you really enjoyed wearing that velvet dress, Mrs. G. You must
have looked lovely."

Using associations as an ancillary technique also provides the
leader with additional information about the patient's life that can
be filed away and used at other times, for example, when the leader
is sitting and chatting with the patient. He may also share this
information with other staff members because these additional
facts may be of help in planning activities and in understanding
choices of friends and general current behavior.

Leadership Techniques

Every group leader eventually develops his own style, but a new
leader needs guidelines. Below we shall discuss some of these
guidelines.

use repetition

Repetition is a most essential part of the total group process and group interaction. Nonverbal repetition is valuable to those who are hard of hearing or whose attention spans are short. Repeating verbal responses permits everyone to share the responses and it also gives feedback to the contributing group member and acts as a reinforcer for the entire group. That is, if the response is repeated often enough, this response has more likelihood of appearing over and over again than if it is not reinforced by repetition.

call the patient by name

The patient's name should be used frequently because it gives recognition to the patient and it reinforces the group and the contributing member to remember the name being verbalized. Therefore, all appropriate verbal and nonverbal responses should be repeated by the leader. Inappropriate responses should be extinguished by not repeating them.

structure the session

Patients should be encouraged to follow the structure of the session strictly. Digressions hinder concentration and take away from the cohesive structure of the group. Comments that do not pertain to the sequence of the session can be dealt with at the end of the session by the leader who may state that fact in a cursory, though receptive way.

move around

The leader should be in constant motion; he should never stand in any one place too long because this decreases the effect of the leader's being the dominant teacher. The leader should move around to each patient as he responds and should stand next to or behind the patient's chair. This prevents the rest of the members from being excluded. Thus, the group is not dominated by just one person, the leader.

touch the patient

Touching is a very essential part of this particular technique. It conveys a feeling of warmth and acceptance to the other person. It says, in effect, "I am here and I care." Touch is a form of communication and reward. Therefore, as the leader moves around the group, he should touch the patients on the shoulder or arm in order to create a warm, accepting atmosphere. When the individual patient responds to the stimulus presented, the leader should touch him and repeat the response the patient has just offered. This helps the other patients focus on who is responding and it serves as a reward that is easily understood by the responding group member.

praise the patient

The leader uses praise as a reward. Each response is recognized by the leader with a comment of "good," "fine," "very nice," or similar form of verbal recognition. In addition, eye contact should be maintained at all times in order to encourage additional responses and to further create a feeling of warmth between the leader and each individual patient.

adjust the tempo of the session

The leader's voice should be loud and clear and he should *speak slowly* and project his voice so that everyone in the group can hear him. The tempo of the session should be slow and smooth. When the leader appears to rush through the session, it may give the group the impression that he wants to get it over with quickly. Older people are slower in responding to stimuli, i.e., slower in processing "input." Therefore, if one of the goals in this technique is to "deconfuse" the environment, rushing through the session may mean that some of the group members are going to miss some aspects of the total group experience.

The leader should also allow ample time for each group member to respond. The total process of receiving sensory stimulation, understanding it or integrating it, and reacting to it in the form of an expressed response takes varying amounts of time. The group member who takes a little longer than others to respond should not be penalized. The leader should understand and work with the differences in response time.

Questions and Answers about Sensory Training

How can a disruptive member be handled? It is very important not to have any disruptions in a primary group. If a member is disruptive, he should be told that he can stay in the group only if he can control his behavior but if he cannot, he will be asked to leave. Sometimes this is enough for change to take place. However, if the patient refuses to be quiet, he should be firmly but kindly escorted out of the session and told that perhaps the next time he will be able to join the group and stay for the whole session. This can be tried for two or three sessions but if there is no improvement, the patient should be dropped from the group. The group must not be sacrificed for the individual.

In a secondary group in which the members are more aware and are more verbal the leader should ask the other patients what they think of the disruptive member's behavior, thus eliciting peer group pressure if it is needed. It has been found that they will usually say that they find it distracting and that the disruptive member should be quiet and listen. Often the patient will yield to this peer group pressure, but if he does not, he should be asked to leave and given the option to return if his behavior improves. This gives him the sense of mastery and choice over his behavior.

If the leader thinks that the disruptive member is capable, he could ask him to act as a co-leader. By leading one of the exercises or helping a less capable member, the disruptive patient receives the attention he craves in a more positive and constructive way.

What about people who do not like to be touched? To most people touching conveys a feeling of warmth and closeness and is usually appreciated. Occasionally, there will be a patient who does not want to be touched. The leader should accept this. A feeling of closeness can be obtained in other ways and the patient should not be ignored. The leader should stand near the patient during the group, perhaps touching the back of the patient's chair. Shaking hands and doing exercises in pairs are more acceptable forms of touching for some people. Gradually, as the group experience progresses, the patient may begin to see touching as a nonthreatening form of communication and may even welcome it.

How are handicapped patients integrated into the group? When a handicapped patient, for example, a blind patient, is brought into the group for the first time, the leader may explain, in detail, what is happening in the group. The blind patient is thus able to both understand and follow the process. The leader can also help the blind patient do the exercises until he become familiar with the routine. When the leader begins the sensory exercises, he explains to the group that the patient is blind and the ramifications of this. When the sight exercise is being performed, the other patients may look at the blind person and describe to him how he looks, what he is wearing at this time, and so on. This is greatly appreciated by the blind person because it enables him to get an image of how he looks and it allows him to interact with his peers. For the other senses, the blind person may be made aware of the fact that these senses are still functioning and that they may help him compensate for the loss of his sight.

Deaf and foreign-speaking patients can be dealt with in a similar fashion. Since the session is very structured and sequential, it is easily understood. Exercises can be imitated with the leader or other patients acting as the model. Verbal responses may not be understood, but facial expressions and mannerisms can be explained by the leader or by the group members.

Doesn't repetition become boring?   The structure of sensory training does not become boring to the patient unless he is on a higher level of functioning, in which case he should be moved to a more demanding group such as reality orientation or remotivation. Repetition offers the patient an opportunity to use his memory, an opportunity to be able to predict events, and an opportunity to develop a sense of mastery. All of this is intended to improve self-confidence. If a patient should become bored, he should either be given more tasks to do or be promoted.

What is the procedure for moving a patient to a higher level group?   As a patient improves and is ready to graduate to a higher level, he should attend both groups for a few sessions and then be gradually dropped from the lower level group. This allows him time to adjust to a new, more demanding group while separating from an old, mastered group.

What is the usual duration of a group?   There is no usual duration. The amount of time that the group continues to meet varies greatly according to the patients, the leader, and the institution. Some patients never progress to a higher group but are able to maintain their functioning in a primary sensory training group. At this point, it is up to the staff and the institution to determine how long the group is to function. The group could function indefinitely. In some institutions the leader works with a group of patients for a specific period of time. If it is seen that some patients are not progressing, they are dropped so that new patients may be afforded the opportunity of a group. In this way, patients who seem to have more potential receive treatment. Sometimes a patient may not respond for a few months, even a year, but then may seem to improve. Each patient should be given ample time in which change may be noted. It has been found that some progress can usually be seen within two to three months.

Should records be kept?   Records of each session should be kept in order to enable the group leader to evaluate progress over time. Each patient's responses to each session should be recorded as soon after a session as possible so that the group leader will not forget any important detail (see Appendix B).

Isn't this technique patronizing to the aged person?   Because of its simplified structure it is often felt that sensory training may be patronizing to the older adult. It is not a patronizing technique however, because the tasks are realistically based on the fact that these patients are extremely regressed. Nonetheless, it is well for the group leader to modify the tone and level to coincide with the patients' backgrounds and abilities. For example, a man who was an engineer might enjoy working with shapes and forms as a means of reidentifying formerly familiar stimuli.

Charting Progress

The best measure of progress is a well-kept record of each session (see Appendix B). By charting a patient's responses immediately after each session the group leader develops an accurate ongoing profile of the patient's behaviors. If well-documented reports are made over a specified period, the patient's progress (or lack of it) will become evident.

    If the leader uses a sensory training evaluation form, he circles the number of the item that corresponds most closely to the patient's response to the task described during that particular session. For example, if the patient was able to identify his body parts sometimes but not always during that session, then "sometimes" or "1" would be the appropriate rating for that patient that day. In addition to rating all the responses to the different program components, ratings are also given to indicate the patient's general level of interest and enjoyment during each session. The leader might also periodically ask other staff if there is any carryover of behavior. When a patient's behavior shows that he is ready for a more advanced group, he should be moved to one. Progress is indicated by the changes in individual item scores (there are no data available on cumulative scores). The evaluation form was developed for the purpose of noting changes in individuals over time. Since there are as yet no norms for what persons should score on this form, its importance lies in its reflecting change. For example, if a patient has been consistently scoring a "1" ("sometimes") on several items and suddenly begins scoring a consistent "2" ("usually"), this is a sign of progress.

The evaluation form is filled out in triplicate after each session[1] (a New York State regulation mandates 30 minutes per week for "Stimulation Techniques"). Although New York and some other states have the 30-minutes-per-week requirement it is not yet federally mandated. One form is placed in the patient's medical chart (usually kept in the nursing station on each unit of each floor); one form is kept by the group leader (to be used after one month with his supervisor), and one form is sent to the chief trainer who may be an occupational therapist, a recreational therapist, or a nurse. At the end of approximately six sessions[2] (groups may have met twice or three times a week, depending on staff duty, trained personnel available, etc.) the leader should meet with his supervisor of training to discuss the patient's progress. They both should examine the particular areas in which the patient has made progress and those in which the patient has declined. When a patient needs additional work, extra sessions should be provided. When a patient shows sufficient progress, "promotion" to a higher level group is suggested.

---

[1]Norms have not yet been established for this technique.

[2]Records can be appraised after six, twelve, or eighteen sessions.

7

reality orientation

Background and Goals

Reality orientation, developed by J. C. Folsom, is an intervention strategy based on repetition and relearning that was developed for use with the moderately confused geriatric patient who is disoriented as to time, place, and/or person. The goal is to heighten the patient's sense of reality by providing him with consistent accurate information about himself and his environment. It started as an aide-centered activity program for elderly patients at the Veterans Administration Hospital in Topeka, Kansas, and went through several refinements, especially at the Veterans Administration Hospital in Tuscaloosa, Alabama.[1]

At that time, many elderly patients were placed in psychiatric facilities for lack of other available services. These patients were relegated to the "back wards" where they received custodial care. Here they suffered the effects of institutionalization, including depersonalization and sensory deprivation. If the patients were not very disoriented on admission, institutionalization often led to increased confusion. With this increased confusion eventually came a nonawareness of time, place, and/or person.

---

[1]L. R. Stephens, ed., *Reality Orientation*, rev. ed. (Washington, D.C.: Hospital and Community Psychiatry Service, American Psychiatric Association, 1975).

Target Population

Reality orientation is a rehabilitation technique offered to the patient who is confused and needs reorienting. It may be appropriate for the patient who suffers from an organic cerebral deficit resulting from organic brain syndrome, a head injury, or a stroke. The patient's confusion may be temporary in some cases and it may fluctuate from day to day.

Composition of the Group

A reality orientation group may consist of members who exhibit a slightly wider range of function than those who are members of "sensory" groups. All reality orientation group members have some verbal skills, although interpersonal skills, i.e., the ability to communicate and interact with others, may vary widely.

Ideally, there should be from three to five patients in a classroom session. However, this number may vary depending on institutional demands such as the number of patients who could benefit from reality orientation and the skills and training of the staff. Modification may, therefore, be determined by the "reality" of the institutional setting.

Time

A time of day for reality classes depends on institutional schedules. The important factor is that the classes are held every day at the same time to encourage a consistent environment. The following should be considered: meal schedules, shift changes, medication times, schedules of various other therapies (e.g., if the physical therapist comes in only from two to four o'clock, this would be an inopportune time for the reality class), staff availability, patient alertness, and receptivity. It should be stressed, however, that the class itself is but one facet of the *total* reality orientation program.

Frequency

Optimally, classroom sessions should be held every day for approximately 30 minutes each time. If this is not possible, sessions should be as frequent as practical, e.g., three times per week. Most importantly, it should be noted that the classroom by itself is not a reality orientation program. In fact, its effectiveness was found to be questionable when there were no facility-wide supports and reinforcements.[2] Moreover, unless the "therapists" who are instructing the classes are adequately trained and supervised on an ongoing basis, the purpose of the classroom may become so distorted that it refutes the assumptions implicit in the reality orientation technique.[3]

In a reality orientation program the teaching process goes on 24 hours a day on a continuous basis. Information pertaining to name, time, and place can be reviewed several times during each day, e.g., while the patient is grooming, at mealtimes, at the start of an occupational therapy or activities program, and so on.

Place

The group should meet consistently in the same place every time. The room should be comfortable, well lit, and free of distractions. The arrangement of chairs depends on the number of participants and the use of various props, e.g., a reality board, a blackboard, etc. Provision must be made for including wheelchairs in the seating arrangement. Ideally, patients should be seated in a circle, but this, of course, may not always be feasible. If no separate room is available, sessions may be conducted on the wards or even in a patient's room.

Materials for Reality Orientation

Suggested materials for use around the facility include large, attractive clocks, calendars and bulletin boards, seasonal decorations, tray favors, and patient and staff name tags.

Suggested classroom materials include individual calendars, word-letter games, blackboard, feltboard, various building block devices for coordination and color matching, plastic numbers, large-piece puzzles, and a reality orientation board.

---

[2] J. A. Barnes, "Effects of Reality Orientation Classroom on Memory Loss, Confusion and Disorientation in Geriatric Patients," *The Gerontologist* **14** (1974): 138–142.

[3] J. R. Gubrium and M. Sander, "Multiple Realities and Reality Orientation," *The Gerontologist* **15** (1975): 142–145.

Reality Orientation Board

The reality orientation board (Fig. 7.1) may be made by using a
wooden board with slots. Words are printed on strips of cardboard.
The words are then slipped into the slots. Fixed above the slots may
be headings such as the name of this place (the answer, the name of
the institution, either remains stationary or is slid into place once

NAME OF INSTITUTION	
THE YEAR IS	19 _ _
TODAY IS	Thursday
THE DATE IS	January 14
THE NEXT MEAL IS	Supper
THE WEATHER IS	Rainy
THE NEXT HOLIDAY IS	Lincoln's Birthday

Figure 7.1 Basic set-up of a reality board for classroom use. (One
should be present in the classroom and, if possible, in day rooms.)

the group member has identified the name); the year; the date
(here a group member is asked the date; if the answer is correct, the
date is placed on the board); the day (same as preceding); the next
holiday is; the weather today is (here words such as "cloudy,"
"sunny," "rainy," or "windy," are affixed to the board); the last
meal was (here the meal that was last eaten is affixed to the board);
the next meal to be eaten (same as in preceding), etc. It has been
found that the board may be modified depending on the needs of
the patients and the demands of the environment. The topics may
range from the simple to the moderately sophisticated (see Fig.
7.2). Every session should include the use of the reality board. This
and similar boards should be posted on every floor because they
help to orient not only the group participants but also the general
patient population. (In one facility the more intact patients were
observed using the board when writing letters or sending greeting
cards because the board offered them needed information.)

WARD ____

Today is	Sunday, Monday, Tuesday, and so on
The date is	January, February, December, and so on 1 to 31
The year is	19 ___
The weather is	hot, cold, warm, cloudy, sunny, rainy, snowy, foggy, clear, humid, and so on
The next holiday is	New Year's day
	Lincoln's birthday
	Washington's birthday
	St. Patrick's day
	Easter
	Passover
	Mother's day
	Memorial day
	Father's day
	Independence day
	Labor day
	Columbus day
	Veteran's day
	Halloween
	Thanksgiving day
	Chanukah
	Christmas
	Martin Luther King's birthday

Figure 7.2   A detailed reality-orientation board.

Refreshments as Reinforcers

Below is an example of how refreshments may be used as part of the program.

Therapist:	[*standing in front of Mary and holding an apple*] Mary, what is this?
Mary:	I don't know.
Therapist:	[*hands apple to Mary*] What color is it?
Mary:	It's red.
Therapist:	That's right, Mary. It's red, and it's something to eat.
Mary:	We do?
Harry:	It's an apple.
Therapist:	That's right, Harry. Did you hear that, Mary? It's an apple. Now, let's all taste our apples. . . .

As with sensory training, refreshments may be used as reinforcers. How and where refreshments are used (at the end of the program or as an incentive to attend) depends on the structure of the program set up by the leader. It has been found, however, that it is most useful to serve refreshments at the conclusion of a program while the leader is informing the group about the next session.

Written Schedule

It is advisable to post the schedule of sessions as well as a list of participants in as many conspicuous areas as possible. Perhaps the written schedule could be attached to the reality boards.

The Leader

The leader should be someone who has been specially trained in the techniques of reality orientation. Although persons from different disciplines may have been trained in this area, direct-care persons such as nursing aides have been most actively involved in conducting reality orientation sessions. The leader should be calm, patient, and empathic. In this technique the leader functions more as a teacher than does the sensory training leader. In the reality orientation classroom value is placed on the correctness of the patient's response, for this group is less regressed and is capable of producing correct responses. Therefore, the leader must encourage accurate responses and offer reinforcement in the form of praise for each right answer, for example, he would say, "Good," "That's fine," or "You are right, Mrs. Jones."

In order to maintain an atmosphere of consistency, the leader should remain with the same group as much as possible. Provision for a consistent replacement such as a co-leader should be made for vacation and sick time. Whenever possible, the group should know the co-leader and be told of the replacement in advance. The purpose of this is to establish and maintain a continuous tie with the leader figure. This tie has been found to be a critical factor in the success of an approach or treatment. When this link is disrupted, for example, when a new leader replaces the old, the total functioning of the group may suffer. This disruption may cause the patients to regress, hostility toward the new group leader, a decrease in attendance, and an increase in expressed bodily ills. However, once the new leader, if he becomes the official replacement, is accepted as *the* leader, the above signs may vanish until the next new leader enters the scene.

Role of the Leader During the Session

The leader is responsible for establishing a warm, congenial atmosphere. He should be accepting and empathic. He should be aware of his gestures, voice, and manners and use them for the benefit of the group members. When he speaks, he should speak in a loud, clear, easily understandable voice. His sentences should be short, direct, and uncomplicated in order to make contact with each patient.

Although the leader should correct inaccurate responses offered by a group member, his manner should in no way indicate disapproval of the group member himself. The group member should be made to feel accepted at *all times* regardless of the "rightness" or "wrongness" of his answer. Each member should be encouraged to offer a correct response but he should not be made to feel guilty or ashamed when he does not respond correctly. This unqualified acceptance of the group member by the group leader helps bring about a heightened sense of self-continuity and self-esteem, which are the essential components and prime goals of all the treatment approaches.

Twenty-Four Hours of Reality Orientation

Reality orientation is a two-pronged program. It is conducted in
the general institution where signs, clocks, calendars, menus, and
so on, identify for the patient the date, place, hour, room, the meal,
and the activity. Above all, the individual is constantly reminded of
his name. His bed and belongings have his name on them. He is
always addressed by his name. He is also always reminded of the
name of the person to whom he is talking. The orientation to reality
goes on during *all* of the patient's waking hours. The patient is
continuously reminded of *who* he is, *where* he is, *why* he is here, and
what is expected of him. In other words, a *twenty-four-hour reality
orientation* is put into effect in order to maintain a total atmosphere
of consistency.

In contrast, the structured reality orientation classes are
carried out in designated areas selected for convenience by staff
personnel. If possible, the classes meet for an intensive 30 minutes
each day. If this is not possible, modification may be made.

Reality orientation sessions need not be as rigidly ordered as
sensory training sessions because the material to be covered
depends very much on the patient's mastery of the information
presented. At each session the leader presents current information
over and over—the patient's name, where he is, the date, etc. As the
patient progresses, additional information may be introduced
(age, home town, occupation, family, etc.).

Each session begins with learning names, for example:

Leader:	Good morning, Mr. Smith. I am Mr. Jones.
	[*Leader repeats his name if necessary.*]
	I am Mr. Jones.
Mr. Smith:	Good morning, Mr. Jones.
Leader:	Good, Mr. Smith. Do you know the lady who is sitting next to you?
	[*Mr. Smith shrugs.*]
Leader:	Mr. Smith, this is Mrs. Silvers. . . .

Or at another session:

Leader:	Good morning, Mrs. Hall. I'm glad you could come today.
Mrs. Hall:	I've got to get to work.

Leader:	What work, Mrs. Hall?
Mrs. Hall:	I'm a teacher.
Leader:	Are you a teacher now?
Mrs. Hall:	Yes.
Leader:	Do you feel well enough to work now?
Mrs. Hall:	No.
Leader:	Mrs. Hall, you are here, at Wayne Rest Nursing Home because you haven't been feeling well and aren't able to work.
Mrs. Hall:	Here? Where? Who are you?

The leader should next provide simple activities, such as identifying pictures, reading the reality orientation board, writing his name, and doing simple manipulative activities. Suggested classroom materials include individual calendars, word-letter games, blackboard, feltboard, mock-up clock, various building block-type devices for coordination and color matching, plastic numbers, large-piece puzzles, and a reality orientation board.

Innovations in Technique:
Using Associations

Some leaders have found that in addition to using familiar objects (a bowl of fruit) associations to the items are helpful. For example, a female patient may be identifying an apple in a bowl of fruit. She may be holding it and gently stroking it. It may be helpful to ask, "Mrs. Smith, what does the apple remind you of?" She may say, "I used to make applesauce at home." The leader could then say, "Yes, applesauce is made from apples. I'll bet you were a good cook. What else did you make?" This kind of dialogue may encourage patients to associate the current experience with some meaningful event in the past. It helps memory by reinforcing memory traces and it gives additional significance to the experience they are now sharing in the group. It is also a way for the leader and other group members to share in some of the experiences in the patient's earlier life and through them to know the patient better. It has been found that association moves the group experience beyond "children's play," sometimes referred to by patients. Association adds new dimensions.

In addition to using everyday objects, the leader may also

introduce a mirror and ask the patient to look at it and report what she sees. Often the responses to the image in the mirror are negative, for example, "I see only an old face with wrinkles" or "What's to see?" as she pushes the mirror away, or "I see someone about 30 years old." All of these responses reveal the "anguish over the stigmata of old age."[4] When a patient gives a negative response when she looks in the mirror, another group member may be asked to tell the group how she sees the person who is holding the mirror. Often the second group member's response is a positive one (i.e., "I see Mrs. Smith looking nice") and can be used to change the faulty perceptions of the one who is looking in the mirror. Additional positive responses can be elicited from the group. In this way the viewing member is confronted with the fact that others see her as, for example, "an old lady with a very pretty face and smile," "a lady with nice coloring and wisdom lines in her face," etc. This technique is used to induce the viewing member to accept old age and correct her misperceptions of herself.

Associations may be used with other events in the person's life. For example, the group member may be asked to look at paintings in the room, describe them, and relate them to paintings, drawings, or prints he may or may not have had in his own home. They may help remind him of past times, family, and friends of the past. Past and present are thus linked within the therapeutic process.

Family Involvement in Reality Orientation

Family members should be included in the overall treatment plan whenever possible. This technique promotes the continuity and consistency of the treatment. When a patient is involved in a reality orientation class and when a consistent attitude is maintained by staff all day, it is harmful to have family members disrupt the reality orientation. They want to be "nice" and not "disturb mama," but they encourage mama's nonreality-oriented statements. Therefore, family members should be taught not to agree with the patient's disoriented statements but to give the patient reality information at all times. For example, a patient may be holding a doll in her arms and referring to it as a baby, pretending that it is alive and treating it as a baby. It has been found helpful to suggest to the patient that the item she is holding is a doll but that she wishes

---

[4]M. Oberleder, "Crisis Therapy in Mental Breakdown of the Aging," *The Gerontologist* **10** (1970): 111–114.

it were a baby. It may be further suggested to her that her wish is based on her own need to have something to cuddle and hold next to herself, a need to have something she can call exclusively her own. In this way, although reality is introduced and she is definitively told that the item is a doll and *not* the baby she perceives it to be, her wishes are interpreted. This is done with warmth, empathy, and with no attempt to take the doll away from her. She is allowed to hold it although it is always referred to realistically, i.e., the *doll* is a *doll.* The patient's family should be told how staff handles this situation and it should be suggested that the family do the same.

It is further suggested that encouraging the patient's disoriented statements is demeaning to the patient and that suggesting that "it is all right to be confused" is in contradiction to the stated goals of therapeutic programs which are to provide reality for the patient. When the family members are encouraged to be part of the treatment, they are usually very supportive and become important members of the reality team. They should be informed of the patient's progress whenever possible so that they may share more directly in that progress.

Reality Orientation Technique: General Points for the Leader

use repetition

Begin each session with a review of the basic information. The leader cannot over-review since reality orientation is based on repetition and relearning. If a patient is unable to give the desired response, the leader should give him the answer and ask him to repeat it. When a patient has difficulty in verbal expression, he should be asked to write a response or express himself in other ways, e.g., use anagrams, scrabble cubes, or magnetic letters on a board. In other words, the leader must be flexible and creative enough to use alternative means when the usual procedures prove inadequate.

establish attainable goals

The leader should not expect too much from patients in reality orientation at first. The activities to be used in reorienting the patient are simple: identifications of familiar objects, picture recognition, word pictures, and the matching and repetition of simple information. These form the basis of the program. The leader must remember that the activity itself is not the only essential ingredient. That is, the activity should lend itself to simple, friendly conversation. It is the friendly, familiar conversation that builds self-confidence for the patient.

If the patient seems aware of the basic information (on the reality board that the leader uses as a prop), he should then be asked about such things as his home town, his family, his former occupation, etc. The leader should know the accuracy of these answers. Thus, it is essential that the reality orientation leader be familiar with the background and history of each patient.

reinforce the right answer

The patient should be rewarded *immediately* after a correct response. The leader should say "good," "that's right," or "fine." If a patient does not give the correct response, the leader should tell him the correct response and ask him to repeat it before the leader moves on. Praise, small rewards (refreshments), and special favors should be used to increase learning.

maintain coordination

It is suggested that at the inception of the program someone be designated as the team leader. This could be the activities worker, a staff nurse, a group worker, an aide, or an orderly. The team leader must be thoroughly familiar with both staff and patients and must have the time to devote to making the program work. He must be responsible for maintaining an ongoing program of in-service training and evaluation of reality orientation. When there is staff turnover, the team leader must be responsible for orienting new staff and integrating them into the team.

In order to get the program underway, outside resources might be used. (The Veterans Administration Hospital at Tuscaloosa has various training programs and state departments of health and state nursing home associations may be able to provide consultation and training.)

In addition to the benefits that will accrue to the patients, increased staff involvement in reality orientation, as in any therapeutic process, tends to produce an increase in staff morale.

Increased staff morale is part of the beneficial aspects of an environment conducive to overall patient improvement.

Integration of Reality Orientation into the Institutional Routine

Again, it must be stressed that reality orientation is more than a classroom exercise on a time-limited basis. Instead, it is an ongoing, total thrust that must be integrated into the environment on a *twenty-four-hour basis.* The following suggestions are offered:

1. All staff should call all patients by their surnames and by their correct titles (Mr./Mrs./Miss/Ms.) unless a patient specifically requests the use of his first name.

2. It is extremely important that staff *know* each patient, especially his social history (family make-up, former occupation, place of birth, etc.), so that appropriate information can be reinforced in casual contacts and conversations.

3. There should be many clocks, calendars, and bulletin boards to heighten the patients' awareness of time, place, and events.

4. There should be an interesting, diversified program of activities appropriate not only to time and place but also in keeping with individual patient needs and interests.

5. The public address system, if available, should be used daily to remind patients of the day, time, and place. An example would be:

Activities worker: Good morning. Today is Thursday, March 21. It's a sunny, spring-like day. This morning we are having the first meeting of our Garden Club at ten o'clock in the lounge. That's one-half hour from now—ten o'clock in the lounge.

6. The dining room should have name cards and patients should be encouraged to behave realistically, i.e., to be considerate of others, to use appropriate utensils. An example would be:

Aide: [*After seeing patient eating with knife.*] Mr. Smith, here's your fork for eating the meat and the peas and potatoes on your plate. Shall I butter the bread with the knife?

7. Appropriate meals should be served on special holidays not only because this is a nice, pleasant gesture; it is also a reality vehicle.

8. Birthdays should be recognized individually by giving the patient a corsage, card, basket, or individual cake (this is in addition to the collective monthly birthday party). The birthday is a vehicle of reality. It also adds a "homey" touch.

9. Clearly written, attractive activities schedules (weekly, biweekly, or monthly) should be given to each resident because they help the patient differentiate the days.

10. Visiting hours should be liberal because they encourage contact with family and friends and tend to help keep patients in touch with reality. However, a word of caution here: Again, family members must be informed about the consistent attempt to keep patients oriented and they must be requested to assist by not reinforcing patients' delusional, hallucinatory, or regressed material. For example, if mother says, "I want to go upstairs to the bedroom now," her daughter should not say, "Okay, mother" to appease her but, rather, "Mother, you are here at Wayne Nursing Home and we are sitting right here in your room."

11. Good contact should be maintained with the community:

(a) Volunteers should be instructed, the same as staff, regarding the infusion of reality into all facets of the nursing home.

(b) Community groups should not only entertain the resident but should also keep the resident in contact with the outside world.

12. Because of the high incidence of visual impairment, color should be used to differentiate one room from another, one door from another, one hallway from another, etc.

13. There should be adequate lighting. Lighting is extremely important in keeping people oriented. Dim lights often discourage environmental contact. Similarly, glare can be a problem, e.g., glare on hallway floors can be frightening and even disorienting.

14. The home should be cheerfully decorated at all times and the decorations should be appropriate to the season. Patients should be encouraged to keep some memorabilia, e.g., pictures of grandchildren, mementos of past trips or achievements, and staff should be instructed to take note of these.

15. Independence should be encouraged. Patients should be expected to dress and groom themselves as much as is practicable. If a patient does need assistance, an aide should do these things *with* the patient rather than *for* him. Whenever appropriate, adapted equipment should be used to maintain independence, e.g., special utensils for hemiplegics, longhandled combs, zipper pulls, etc.

16. Whenever practicable, more than one sense should be stimulated. For example, in activities programs the patient may receive input visually through the written activities schedules and auditorially when the aide comes to the room and talks to the patient to encourage him to attend.

Questions and Answers about Reality Orientation

Administratively, how does one go about introducing a reality orientation therapy program? First, there must be a commitment from the top. If this is to be a total thrust, everybody must participate, i.e., every staff member, including office and maintenance personnel, volunteers, and even family. It does not take long to discover that *attitudes are caught, not taught.* Before any commitment can be made, one has to honestly assess his facility and determine what modifications might be made to initiate or to increase the reality thrust. Essentially, what is involved here is an attitudinal commitment instead of a financial commitment.

What is "reality" for the nursing home patient? What difference does it make if it is Tuesday and not Friday? Nobody is going any place anyway. But, Tuesday should be different from Friday! When the reality orientation technique was originally conceived, it was for elderly mental hospital patients. Some of these patients progressed so well that they were assigned to other therapies, e.g., remotivation, occupational therapy, music therapy, speech therapy, physical therapy, group therapy, etc., and eventually were discharged into the community. But many of today's institutionalized patients are confined because there is no place for them to go in the community. So, if we restore them to a more optimum level of functioning, what then? This negativism has to be overcome. More emphasis must be placed on the *quality of life within the nursing home or facility.*

Does reality orientation therapy create a "better patient"?
If a "good" patient is a passive-dependent patient, the answer is no.
Reality orientation tends to make the patient more aware of
himself and his environment. The goal is to eventually involve him
in his environment and make *him responsible* for *his behavior.* The
patient is encouraged to again become as independent as possible.
In one study a Ward Behavior Inventory (WBI) was used as a
premeasure and postmeasure of performance to monitor a
comprehensive program of sensory stimulation in a nursing home.
After the program had run for several months, the WBI showed an
increase in disturbed behavior. When the authors examined what
constituted "disturbed," they realized that the renewed
environmental interest had fostered some aggressiveness and
argumentativeness.[5] Although these behaviors might have
indicated greater disturbance in a mental hospital setting, they
truly indicated a successful thrust here because the goal was, in fact,
to get the patients more in touch with their environment.

Is the classroom situation too kindergarten-like?   It must
always be remembered that reality orientation is for the regressed
patient. Some of the items used may well resemble materials that
are used to teach children, e.g., the large mock-up clock. However,
many patients do have, in addition to their general regression, real
sensory impairments that dictate using special materials. If vision is
poor, large numbers are essential; for the highly distractable, there
must be a clear, legible number at every spot. Although care must
be taken that the materials used are not juvenile, realism must be
used in making the necessary adaptations to meet patient needs.
Under no circumstances should the geriatric patient be
infantilized. Indeed, although the structured reality classroom is a
simulated formal learning experience for the regressed patient,
the principle of reality orientation is one that should be practiced
with all patients throughout any institution as a technique of
prevention as well as *intervention.*

Advanced Reality Orientation

Once patients have completed the basic classes, they should be
advanced into the higher level reality orientation classes. The same
procedures that are used in basic classes are used in the advanced

---

[5]C. A. Loew and B. M. Silverstone, "A Program of Intensified Stimulation and
Response Facilitations for the Senile Aged," *The Gerontologist* 11 (1971): 341–347.

classes. The patients are expected to read and copy the reality orientation board and the materials listed on the blackboard. In addition, they are provided with other materials to read and other projects to complete under the advisement of the group leader. Here, spelling, writing, and some simple arithmetic problems may be used. Other activities that may be used include reading and discussing current events, filling in blank quizzes, etc. Discussions may center around any topic of interest to the group. Whenever possible, a group member should be asked to prepare a simple discussion for the group. The emphasis should still be on reality orientation and, thus, whenever appropriate, the days of the week, the time, the date, the name of the place, etc., should be mentioned.

The group leader should introduce himself at each session and welcome each group member by name and with a personal comment on the group member's appearance such as, "How nice your hair looks today, Mrs. Smith" or "I see you have a new haircut, Mr. Armstrong."

Charting Progress

In order to determine when the patient is ready to move onto another, more advanced technique, it is essential to keep progress notes on each session. These records are to be attended to *immediately* after each session in order to allow for the least amount of memory loss on the part of the group leader. The record (see Appendix C) may be modified according to the patients in the leader's group or the ingenuity or flexibility of the leader. The essential point is that some record of each patient's progress be kept in order to know when and if progress has taken place. The form is filled out in *triplicate,* one for the medical chart (placed there at the end of a month), one for the group leader, and one for the group leader's supervisor.

It is suggested that a record be kept for each patient for each session. Progress is indicated by consistent improvement on overall scores.[6] Although there may be progress in one area, e.g., verbal communication, other item scores may tend to remain the same. This is not to be taken as a sign of lack of improvement since improvement will not necessarily be consistent for all items.

At the end of the six-week series, the leader should meet with his supervisor to discuss each patient's progress. At this point, decisions are made about promoting the patient, continuing him in

---

[6]Norms have not yet been established for this technique.

the same group, providing additional supportive measures, etc. Records should be appraised after six, twelve, or eighteen sessions, depending on the decision of the leader and the realities of the environment.

Attitude Therapy: An Adjunct Therapy with Reality Orientation

Attitude therapy is usually used in conjunction with reality orientation. Basically, each patient's style of behavior is first identified. Then the staff decides upon and prescribes a staff style of behavior, i.e., an attitude toward this patient. The patient is treated *consistently* with *all* staff members relating to him in the same way. The five basic attitudes are active friendliness, passive friendliness, matter-of-fact, kind firmness, and no demand. These five attitudes tend to reinforce those behaviors that are adaptive for the patient and not reinforce those that are maladaptive. Although attitude therapy was developed as an adjunct to reality orientation, it may be used as a general approach to the patient. That is, a consistent way of relating to a patient based on his habitual style of responding to the environment is appropriate regardless of the level of functioning of the patient and/or whether or not he is engaged in any specific treatment modality.

active friendliness

Active friendliness is to be used with the apathetic, withdrawn patient. The staff should seek out the individual who is withdrawn and has little or no confidence in himself and attempt to counteract this patient's feelings of failure. As J. C. Folsom describes it, this patient must be "loved back to health."[7] An example follows:

> Mr. E., a man in his late 80's sits in his room all day. The only time spent out of his room is to eat in the dining room only remaining there for a few minutes at each meal. He has no confidence in himself and cannot even say if he feels good. All of his statements are laden with the words: "maybe"; "I guess so"; "I don't really know"; etc.[8]

For him, the staff exhibits an attitude of active friendliness. For example, after this type of patient has shaved, staff could say, "How nice you look" or compliment him on his choice of an article of clothing. Such constructive statements may help rebuild his confidence and trust in himself. Once this trust has been re-established, he can again begin to communicate meaningfully with others around him and improve his overall level of functioning.

passive friendliness

This attitude is used with the frightened, suspicious patient. Here the worker should show interest and concern but should wait for the patient to make the first move. An active approach by staff would only tend to alienate this individual more and should be avoided because friendly gestures may be misinterpreted and may increase the patient's "natural" suspiciousness. An example follows:

> A man, Mr. C., is in his early 60's and confined to a wheelchair. He is overly suspicious of everyone. When someone walks into his room his first thought is: I wonder what he is doing here; what does he want, etc.[9]

The staff approach should be one that indicates that "we are here to help you; we understand; if you want anything, let us know." Here the individual is given the opportunity to take the initiative. Thus, the patient should be encouraged to attend the class, but staff should not insist that he attend the class.

matter-of-fact

The goal here is to help the patient learn to take responsibility for his own behavior. Here the staff is open but "matter-of-fact" with the individual. This attitude is best used with the highly manipulative person or the person who shows social maladjustment in his behavior. Here staff has to be expressly clear that they are *not* to be manipulated and that this behavior will not be rewarded. It is hoped that through this attitude by staff the patient will be able to begin a constructive life pattern. A typical situation follows:

---

[9]Ibid., p. 313.

Mr. M., a man in his late 70's, has the marked characteristic of manipulating members of the staff for cigarettes. Mr. M., because of his smoking habit, age, and physical condition, does not eat.[10]

Once a matter-of-fact attitude is begun and Mr. M. knows that he cannot go from one member of the staff to another to get cigarettes, he will become aware if he wants to enjoy his smoking, he must first accept the fact that he must first eat. It has been found that this kind of person, often avoided by others because of his manipulative behavior, becomes more socially accepted.

kind firmness

This attitude is to be used with the depressed patient. The goal here is to help the patient focus away from himself and to engage him in interaction with others. It is helpful to have this person understand that he may express strong feelings appropriately, such as anger. For example, if the patient is unwilling to get out of bed, it has been found helpful to insist that he get out of bed. An example follows: Mrs. G., a patient who shows depressed behavior, lies in bed and refuses to get up, toilet herself, or get dressed. The worker, upon entering the room, may say, "Mrs. G., you will have to get up and get dressed now. I will wait here for you and help you if you like. Then we will both walk down to the dining room for lunch. You must get up now."

no demand

This attitude is to be used with the frightened, angry patient who is acting out his fears. He may even be in a panic state in which the only way he knows how to act is by showing aggression toward everyone around him and toward himself. The goal of the prescribed attitude of no demand is to remove pressure from the patient while letting him know that nobody is going to harm him. The staff should also let the patient know that they will not respond to his anger. The only rules set down for him are as follows:

1. He cannot leave the treatment area.
2. The staff will not permit him to harm himself.
3. He cannot harm others.
4. He must take his medications.

---

[10]Ibid., p. 317.

Once the person is in control, he should be given positive rewards and positive responses by staff.

Questions and Answers about Attitude Therapy

Who prescribes the attitude to be used?　The appropriate attitude may be selected by the team members on the basis of their knowledge of the patient and their observation of his behavior. It may sometimes be helpful to use a consulting psychiatrist or psychologist, particularly when the patient's behavior does not seem clear to the team members, e.g., the patient is *both* withdrawn and suspicious or agitated *and* depressed.

What is the essential point of attitude therapy?　The essential point is consistency. Each staff member should use the same approach in *all* his interactions with the patient. The patient should then be able to understand what is expected of him and to respond accordingly. In some facilities prescribed attitudes are made apparent to staff by the use of color-coded name tags. For example, pink may mean the attitude of active friendliness and green may mean the attitude of matter-of-fact. These colors may be posted on the door of the patient's room, his bed, or any other obvious place.

What are the most commonly used attitudes in conjunction with reality orientation?　The usual attitudes in the reality class are active friendliness and passive friendliness. No matter what, the instructor must be supportive. The demands are minimal. As soon as the patient responds, he should be rewarded with praise. When a patient has mastered even the most simple task, his accomplishments should be made known to the entire team. Repetition, in both words and in writing, is the keystone. Social interaction with other members of the class should be constantly encouraged.

Can the prescribed attitude change?　The prescribed attitude is subject to change depending on changes in the patient's mode of behavior. That is, should a patient become ill and suddenly become withdrawn and apathetic during the early recovery period, the staff would then adopt an attitude of active friendliness even though the prescribed attitude for this patient may have been any one of the other attitudes. It is recommended that the patient's progress be noted and reviewed periodically.

Who does attitude therapy?   There is no special "attitude therapist." It is suggested that every staff member practice this technique for it cannot be emphasized too often that *consistency* is the key to patient progress.

remotivation technique

A patient is promoted to remotivation when it has been determined by staff that he is ready for this therapeutic intervention. It may also happen that an alert patient who has never evidenced a need for sensory training or reality orientation therapy may be assigned directly to remotivation as the modality best suited to him.

Background and Goals

The remotivation technique was established over 20 years ago by the late Dorothy Hoskins Smith of Claremount College, California, as a remotivator for mentally disturbed patients. It has since been found to be helpful for use with the more alert patients in institutions. Remotivation is a technique of simple group interaction of an objective nature designed to help patients toward reality.[1] The two therapeutic aims considered most essential are as follows:

1. To stimulate patients into thinking about and discussing topics associated with the real world.
2. To assist patients to relate to and communicate with other people.[2]

---

[1] E. K. Barns, A. Sack, and H. Shore, "Guidelines to Treatment Approaches." *The Gerontologist* **13** (1973): 513–527.

[2] Ibid., p. 518.

Initially, it was thought that the personnel who work with this group of aged should be professionals. It was soon found that the technique was one easily learned by the direct-care workers (aides and orderlies) because they were the ones who had the most contact with the patients. It also allowed for the direct-care workers to develop and maintain an increased sense of self-esteem in that they were now active and contributing members of the therapeutic team.

Target Population

Remotivation is appropriate for the patient who, although more alert, still needs a structured vehicle for socialization. This patient is more verbal than those who are in sensory training or reality orientation and is capable of participating, to an extent, in a group discussion. His attention span is also slightly longer. There may be memory deficits, especially in recent memory, e.g., he may not remember what he ate for breakfast, but he can discuss topics that are familiar to and of interest to him, e.g., holidays, sports, fashions, etc. This patient needs structure in the form of clear and consistent expectations and time-limited activities.

Composition of the Group

A remotivation group consists, optimally, of from 10 to 15 patients. Hopefully, a few of these patients will be more advanced than the others and serve as stimulators and "sparkers." Conversely, one or two slightly confused residents may also be included.

It has been found that some leaders prefer smaller groups. This depends on both the needs and abilities of the group members as well as on the group leader. In addition, space limitations and other reality factors should be considered.

Unlike sensory training and reality orientation that allow for "regressed" behavior, remotivation demands a higher level of cognitive functioning and more social interaction. When a patient does exhibit behavior that is disruptive to this group, he must be removed until he is again ready for this form of intervention.

Time

Remotivation sessions should be held once or twice a week and it is advisable that they be held at the same time each week in order to maintain consistency. A word of caution is due here: Scheduling remotivation may be more difficult since these patients are, indeed, capable of participating in a wide range of activities. It is conceivable that an early evening meeting, e.g., after dinner, may be best because other activities are not usually available then.

Frequency

A remotivation program usually consists of a series of 12 sessions held once or twice a week. Each session may require from 30 minutes to an hour, depending on the needs of the group.

Place

The room where the sessions take place should be comfortable, well lit, and as free of distraction as possible. The furniture arrangements should allow for the inclusion of wheelchair patients. When the weather permits, it is possible to conduct remotivation sessions out of doors.

A Written Schedule

Remotivation meetings should be well publicized. They should, of course, be included on a regular activities schedule. In addition, notices should be posted in conspicuous places, for example, on bulletin boards, along the corridors, and in the activities room.

The Remotivator

The discussion leader, referred to as a *remotivation technician,* is one who has attended a 30-hour course in remotivation technique at a training center or nearby hospital where such courses are often given. He should be more formal in his total approach than the leader of the sensory training class or the leader of the reality orientation class because the remotivation technique was devised to simulate a classroom situation, i.e., it is more didactic than the previously described approaches. It adheres to a rigid, precise format and requires advance preparation by the leader who should feel comfortable in this formal setting. He should enjoy discussion, have a good general fund of information, and be able to follow the structured five steps that will be described later.

role of the leader in the session

In many ways, remotivation is similar to a classroom situation in which there is a teacher (the leader) and students (geriatric patients). The leader must be in control of each meeting from start to finish. In fact, it is he who opens and closes the meeting in a very prescribed fashion. It has been found that leaders who followed the structured order of the five steps are more successful than those who do not. The only flexibilities allowed the leader are the length of the steps within each of the sessions and the choice of subject matter. (After several sessions have been conducted, it is sometimes helpful to have a patient choose a topic on which the group agrees and have the patient conduct the session as a leader.)

materials for remotivation

Props for remotivation sessions are readily available, for example, jewelry, hats, shoes, clothing, flowers, pine cones, acorns, and leaves. Other props may be obtained from the dietary department (bread, cake, fruits, jellies, cooking utensils, beer, wine). Other items such as decorations, quilts, and handmade articles may be borrowed from the occupational or activities therapy departments and tools and cleaning utensils may be obtained from the maintenance department. Sometimes it is helpful to ask staff or volunteers who travel on vacation to bring back souvenirs that can be used in the remotivation sessions. In this way, items such as Mexican hats, grass skirts, lava rock, mineral stones, gourds, wine bottles, decorated eggshells, foreign coins, and fancy menus may be collected. Interesting newspaper and magazine articles should be clipped for possible use. In addition, libraries may be used for reference materials as well as films, filmstrips, records. Props and other materials should be properly stored for periodic use and reuse.

Technique

The remotivation technician selects topics recommended in manuals published by the American Psychiatric Association/Smith

Kline & French Remotivation Project.[3] It has been suggested that the topics selected deal with the real world. For example, one could include the history of stamps in our country, presidents, fashions, holidays, or sports. Sensitive (controversial) topics are not usually dealt with.

The following five structured steps should be followed in each remotivation session:

Step I
(3–5 min)

Creating a climate of acceptance. Greet each person by name, shake his hand, make him feel welcome by telling the group that it is good to be with him; establish a warm, congenial ambiance. Say something nice you notice about each individual.

Step II
(5–10 min)

Creating a bridge to reality. Use "bounce" (interest-getting) questions, gradually leading into the subject. Once the topic has been reached, an objective short poem (music, props, displays, and other visual aids may be used) relevant to the topic is read aloud as the remotivator moves around the circle. Any response is accepted by the remotivator who repeats what was said or may reinforce the response with "That's right," "Fine," "Good," etc.

Step III
(15–20 min)

Sharing the world of reality. Using the same type of questions, one develops the topic by asking planned, objective questions. Questions asked are of an "What is . . . How big is . . ." nature. Participants are encouraged to speak to the remotivator and to each other.

Step IV
(15–20 min)

Appreciating the work of the world. The aim here is to stimulate reminiscence and the sharing of experiences, ideas, and opinions which have past, present, and possibly future interest for participants. This is accomplished by investigating the work involved with the topic, the value of that work, the profit associated with it, what training may be involved in that work, etc.

[3]*Remotivation Technique: A Manual for Use in Nursing Homes* (Washington, D.C.: American Psychiatric Association, n.d.).

Step V   *Creating a climate of appreciation.* The
(3–5 min)   remotivator expresses enjoying having
                          been together and summarizes what was
                          said. He shows appreciation for any
                          contributions made by the members and
                          invites participants to bring poems, songs,
                          newspaper clippings, and other items
                          relevant to the next session. He invites the
                          members to the next meeting and, if
                          possible, gives the date and time of the
                          next session.

The following is a transcribed recording of an actual
remotivation session. The members are 10 females from the ages
of 68 to 91 who live in a residential care setting. The session was
conducted by a nursing aide trained in a 30-hour remotivation
in-service training course.

Remotivation Session   Topic—Quilting

Remotivator: Good morning Mrs. W. Thank you for coming to
                 the meeting. Good morning Mrs. A. I'm happy to
                 see you. Mrs. T, welcome. Thank you for coming to
                 the meeting. Miss M, so nice to have you come to our
                 meeting. Mrs. C, I'm glad you could make it. I know
                 it's kind of early to get everybody up. Good morning
                 Mrs. N.

Mrs. N: Mary.

Remotivator: May I call you Mary?

Mrs. N: Oh yes, everybody calls me Mary.

Remotivator: Okay. I'll do that. Good morning Mrs. G. Thank you
                 for coming to the meeting.

Mrs. G: [*Smiles.*]

Miss S: You don't know my name, I bet!

Remotivator: Oh yes, Miss S, and I'm glad you came this morning.
                 Mrs. F, thank you for coming to the meeting.

Mrs. F: Thank you for inviting me.

Remotivator: Mrs. E, it's nice to see you. Thank you for coming.

Mrs. E: I'm glad to be here.

Remotivator: It's kind of warm today, isn't it?

Mrs. G:	It is close, yes.
Remotivator:	What kind of activities does a housewife do in the daytime?
Mrs. A:	Ach du lieber!
Miss S:	Always housework.
Remotivator:	Always housework. Good.
Mrs. T:	Everything.
Remotivator:	Everything. Mrs. T said everything. Mrs. G, what would a housewife do in the daytime?
Mrs. G:	Cleaning, sweeping.
Remotivator:	What did you say Miss S?
Miss S:	Housework.
Remotivator:	Yes. Housework.
Miss M:	Everything.
Remotivator:	That covers a lot of territory!
Miss M:	Yes.
Remotivator:	Mary, what would a housewife do in the daytime?
Mrs. N:	Wash, iron, cooking and . . . wait for your husband to come in.

[Laughter.]

Remotivator:	And wait for your husband to come in. That's true. Mrs. G?
Mrs. G:	Well, she'd start cleaning up the kitchen, the breakfast dishes and all that first.
Remotivator:	Yes. That's right.
Mrs. G:	Then she'd start the luncheon and the dinner . . .
Remotivator:	And get ready for dinner. And how would she keep busy in the evening?
Miss S:	That's dangerous.

[Laughter.]

Remotivator:	That's dangerous?
Miss S:	Washing dishes.

[Laughter.]

Remotivator:	Mrs. F, how would a housewife keep busy in the evening?
Mrs. F:	Sewing, crocheting.
Remotivator:	Sewing, crocheting. Yes. Mrs. E?

Mrs. E:	She cooks supper, turns down the beds . . . listens to the radio.
Mrs. A:	Ya! Ya!
Remotivator:	Oh, she's going to have a nice evening. You are not going to put her to work in the evening? [*Laughter.*] How would a farmwife spend her evening?
Mrs. A:	Take her shoes and run!
Mrs. W:	I know, because I've done it.
Remotivator:	You've done it? What did you do in the evening?
Mrs. W:	Canning.
Remotivator:	Preparing her canning. Is that a lot of work, Mrs. W?
Mrs. W:	As a rule.
Remotivator:	Can anyone else tell me what a farmwife might do in the evening?
Mrs. A:	Begin to despair!
Remotivator:	Oh . . . How did women spend their evenings 60 years ago?
Miss S:	I don't know.
Remotivator:	You don't remember? Miss M, how would a housewife spend her evenings 60 years ago?
Miss M:	Getting ready to go to the theater.
Remotivator:	Yes. She might get ready to go to the theater. How else would a housewife spend her evenings 60 years ago?
Mrs. N:	I was only a baby from my mother. She used to bring me around, and she used to show me a lot of things: cleaning, sewing . . .
Remotivator:	General things?
Mrs. G:	She might get the babies ready for bed and clean up the kitchen and get ready for the morning.
Remotivator:	Yes. All important things.
Miss S:	When my mother finished the work, then she'd go out to her friend's house.
Remotivator:	Go visiting. Yes. . . . Mrs. F, what would you have done 60 years ago?

Mrs. F:	My mother used to wash and iron and catch up for the next day.
Remotivator:	Working and getting ready for the next day. Fine.
Mrs. E:	Sixty years ago my mother, after she got us up to bed, used to get out the carded wool and spin. Each night she'd get out the spinning wheel and warp it up. She'd work every night on that spinning wheel.
Remotivator:	Those were busy evenings. Tell me . . . what kinds of handiwork did women do in a group years ago?
Mrs. E:	In a group?
Remotivator:	Would you know what they did in a group?
Mrs. N:	Make quilts.
Remotivator:	Right. They used to have quilting bees.
Mrs. E:	Oh yes. The quilting bees.
Remotivator:	Did any of you ladies sew in a quilting bee?
Mrs. E:	Oh yes. We did.
Remotivator:	Anyone else?
Mrs. W:	Not in a group. But I did it myself.
Remotivator:	You did it yourself? Did anyone else ever do any sewing in a quilting bee?
Mrs. T:	Mm-Mm-Mm I watched.
Remotivator:	You were just watching it? You didn't do the work? I see. Well, you can know a great deal from watching. . . . Miss M has a poem she'd like to read us on the quilting party.
Miss M:	*The Quilting Party*

In the sky the bright stars glittered
On the bank the pale moon shone,
And it was from Aunt Dinah's quilting party
I was seeing Nellie home.

On my arm a soft hand rested,
Rested light as ocean foam,
And it was from Aunt Dinah's quilting party
I was seeing Nellie home.

[*Applause.*]

Remotivator:	That was very nice Miss M. Thank you. Can anyone tell me what *is* a quilt?

Miss S:	A quilt is a something that starts with pieces of goods like a patchwork and in between the patches, they put cotton.
Remotivator:	They put a cotton padding?
Miss S:	A padding.
Remotivator:	That's right. . . . How else could we describe a quilt?
Mrs. F:	The only thing I know about it is, it is a pretty bedcover.
Remotivator:	Yes. Quilts are bedcovers. And to you Mrs. E, what would you say about a quilt?
Mrs. E;	A bedcover.
Remotivator:	Right.
Mrs. W:	A quilt is a cover made for a bed out of different materials, different sizes, all knitted squares. Also, different sizes . . . and crocheted, too.
Remotivator:	It could be crocheted of any type of materials or wool?
Mrs. W:	That's right.
Remotivator:	Fine. When do you think quilt-making was invented?
Miss S:	Before my time.
Remotivator:	Mrs. C, when do you think quilt-making was invented?
Mrs. C:	Quilt is made of many pieces, putting them together.
Remotivator:	Patching them together. That is a type of quilt. When do you think quilt-making was invented . . . Miss M?
Miss M:	I have no idea.
Miss S:	Before my time.
Remotivator:	Miss S said before her time. Mrs. G, was it before your time?
Mrs. G:	It must have been a long time ago.
Miss M:	At least 70 years ago.
Remotivator:	I read that it probably started in Colonial times, when material was hard to get, so the women used all the little scraps that they had. . . . Can anyone tell me how quilts are made nowadays?
Mrs. F:	They are made by machinery in the factories.

Remotivator:	Yes. They are most often made by machines.
Mrs. N:	We crochet some of them and sew the crocheted pieces together.
Remotivator:	Yes, that is true. . . . Tell me, what different kinds of quilts are there?
Mrs. N:	There's wool. . . .
Mrs. F:	Different kinds of material: wool, cotton; and they put the cotton in between.
Remotivator:	Right. Any other type of quilt that you know? . . .
Mrs. A:	A quilt.
Mrs. C:	Small pieces, put together.
Remotivator:	What would that be called?
Mrs. C:	A quilt.
Remotivator:	There is a special name. Does anyone know what that would be called? Small pieces joined together. What is the name for that type of quilt?
Mrs. E:	A patch quilt.
Remotivator:	A patchwork quilt. That's right, Mrs. E. Are they the easiest ones to make?
Mrs. E:	No. I don't think so.
Mrs. W:	No . . . mm-mm-mm-- Maybe so.
Remotivator:	There is more detail in patchwork quilts, Mrs. W? [*Remotivator picks up small pieces of material.*] I have a few samples here of the materials that are used in making quilts.
Miss M:	Oh, yes.
Miss S:	Calico.
Remotivator:	First you would have just like Miss S says. What is that Miss S? [*Remotivator holds materials and shows them to each in turn.*]
Miss S:	Calico, isn't it? A cotton . . . ?
Remotivator:	A type of cotton. Right.
Mrs. G:	Gingham.
Mrs. F:	A cotton, calico or gingham, more or less.
Remotivator:	Gingham and calico are different types of cotton material. These samples are also types of cotton prints. So you would start with just your materials at first?

Mrs. E:	You collect them.
Mrs. W:	That's bell-shaped.
Remotivator:	That's one design. A bell-shaped design. Yes.
Mrs. A:	[*Looks at it and smiles.*]
Remotivator:	So you collect the pieces. Then what happens after you have your material?
Mrs. T:	Together.
Remotivator:	Put them together, Mrs. T?
Miss M:	Cut it in different sizes, different pieces.
Mrs. N:	You can cut them to the size you want.
Remotivator:	Right. What else can be made of quilted material, besides bedcovers? Now, here's something made from those two pieces of material I showed you. Can you feel the difference? [*Remotivator shows each a set of quilted pot holders made of previously shown materials.*]
Mrs. G:	Yes.
Miss S:	Oh yeah! Pot holders, aren't they?
Mrs. F:	They're made like pants! [*Laughter.*]
Remotivator:	Right . . . And they feel heavier. Is there something in between, or is it just cotton material?
Mrs. E:	This is heavier than that. So there must be something in between, if it is heavier than this one.
Mrs. W:	Let me see.
Mrs. N:	A padding.
Remotivator:	Yes. . . . Mrs. C, can you feel the inside?
Mrs. C:	There's padding inside.
Remotivator:	You're right. You do feel the padding inside?
Mrs. C:	Yes.
Remotivator:	Does all quilting have to have a padding?
Mrs. E:	You could have wool or cotton in layers.
Remotivator:	In layers?
Mrs. E:	Yes. Carded wool or cotton. It's all put in on the frame and they have to put in extra. You have to sit down on a stool and sort it out with your hands.
Remotivator:	You must have had a lot to do in the evenings.

Mrs. E:	Of course we did.
Remotivator:	Can you feel the padding? These are some of the things that were made up in our own therapy department.
Mrs. G:	You can put pieces of cloth in between, or anything . . . rags, if you don't want to save them to wash with.
Remotivator:	That's very interesting. Can you tell me what this is?
	[Shows a quilted mitt with a puppet head.]
Mrs. W:	A cat?
Remotivator:	Yes. It's made to look like a cat.
Mrs. F:	A hot pot mitt!
Mrs. G:	That's what they made.
Remotivator:	A hot pot mitt. . . . Miss S, how do you like this? This was also made in our therapy department.
Miss S:	Something to put on your hand when you get a hot pot?
Remotivator:	Yes. It would be a protection for your hand.
Mrs. G:	I say the same.
Remotivator:	Mrs. A, would you like to put it on?
Mrs. A:	Ya! Ya!
Remotivator:	You would say the same? That's right. Mary?
Miss M:	For your hand on the hot pots.
Mrs. N:	You could use it for everything . . . baking pot, coffee pot, cooking.
Mrs. F:	And your hands would be always good.
Remotivator:	Miss M?
Miss M:	I wouldn't know what it was.
Remotivator:	Would you like to guess?
Miss M:	Some kind of glove.
Remotivator:	Some kind of glove. That's right. Mrs. C?
Mrs. C:	A glove.
Remotivator:	Right. To be used for what?
Mrs. C:	To put on.
Remotivator:	Mrs. T?
Mrs. T:	Mm-mm-mm. Not sure.
Remotivator:	To wear?

Mrs. G:	That's what it looks like: a mitt.
Mrs. T:	Mm-mm-mm. Yes.
Remotivator:	Yes. A mitt. They do these upstairs in the occupational therapy room. Have you seen them work on these upstairs? Mrs. A, would you know what this was?
Mrs. A:	I'm afraid I wouldn't.
Remotivator:	Mrs. W?
Mrs. W:	I can't see the stitches so good. I should imagine it was done by machine?
Remotivator:	Right. This was done by machine upstairs.
Mrs. E:	Isn't it a skull-cap?
Remotivator:	It *looks* like a skull-cap from where you're looking at it. Suppose I put it on my hand?
Mrs. E:	Oh yes.
Remotivator:	. . . But it's a mitten.
Mrs. E:	Oh! That's right.
Remotivator:	. . . To pick up your pots or reach into your oven.
Mrs. W:	I got pot holders I never used.
	[Much simultaneous talking and laughing.]
Remotivator:	Isn't that fancy?
Miss M:	Very fancy.
Miss S:	That looks like a puppet!
Remotivator:	They made these last year. They sold very well. Yes. It's a mitt, made like a puppet. Did you ever use any of these?
	[More talking, laughing.]
Mrs. T:	No.
Mrs. W:	I'm not so sure.
	[Laughter.]
Remotivator:	You didn't like to do any cooking at home?
Mrs. G:	Aah. *[Shrugs.]*
Mrs. A:	*[Looks at remotivator and others, but does not answer, only laughs.]*
Remotivator:	You did and you didn't. Now I have another piece of material here. Sister was nice enough to give us. Mrs. E, you want to feel it?
	[Remotivator shows a large section of an unfinished quilt.]
Mrs. E:	I do. Yes.

Remotivator:	That was what you were talking about?
Mrs. E:	Oh yes. It's like a patch and it's quilted; cut like a quilt.
Remotivator:	That's a quilt. Yes, a portion of it. . . . Mrs. F?
Mrs. F:	Pretty quilting.
Remotivator:	It's nice and soft.
Miss S:	It has cotton in between.
Remotivator:	Yes. It has a cotton in between, that's right.
Miss S:	It's pretty. I'd like this for my bureau.
Remotivator:	You want to take this for your bureau? I'll have to get permission from Sister. All right?
Miss S:	Okay.
Mrs. G:	That's pretty.
Mrs. N:	Like a baby quilt.
Remotivator:	Yes. It's the proper size for a baby's crib.
Mrs. G:	Carriage cover.
Remotivator:	This would be very pretty as a carriage cover . . . Mrs. C?
Mrs. C:	Pretty. Yes.
Miss M:	It is pretty.
Remotivator:	Do you like that?
Mrs. T:	Mm-mmm. Nice.
Remotivator:	Very nice, huh? Want to feel it, Mrs. A? Feel it.
Mrs. A:	Ya!
Remotivator:	See how soft that is.
Miss M:	It is soft.
Remotivator:	Is this what you worked on Mrs. W?
Mrs. W:	No. I didn't do this. I made dresses.
Remotivator:	I see.
Mrs. W:	But I *could* do that.
Remotivator:	You're handy at sewing, I know. . . . Tell me, what color could a quilt be?
Mrs. G:	Any color.
Remotivator:	Yes. Any color. What color would make up prettiest, do you think?
	[*Many responses:* "Blue," "Red," "Pink," "Green," "I like red."]

Remotivator:	Red, blue, pink. You like blue, Mrs. T?
Mrs. T:	Mm-mm-mm. Yes. Blue is nice.
Remotivator:	Miss M?
Miss M:	Depends on the other colors. I don't know.
Remotivator:	According to the color scheme in the room? That's good. Mary, what color quilt would you like?
Mrs. N:	Sounds very good. It could have green, yellow, red, blue. . . .
Remotivator:	What are quilting frames?
Mrs. A:	To curse, huh? [*Laughs.*]
Remotivator:	No. Quilting frames.
Mrs. A:	Oh. I see.
Remotivator:	Do you know what a quilting frame is?
Mrs. A:	No, no, no, I don't. I never did. . . .
Remotivator:	You never did any sewing?
Miss S:	You put the material on them.
Mrs. A:	Yes, I did. [*Laughs.*] I don't want to commit myself.
Remotivator:	All right. Miss S says that the frames are for the quilt material.
Mrs. E:	They're a long piece of wood, dear, and a narrow piece at the ends, and a certain size, and you have to put both threads in and tie them so they pull stiff as you work through.
Remotivator:	To work through. I see. . . .
Mrs. E:	You put the material on them.
Mrs. G:	If it had legs, it could stand up, if it had to be put on the floor. I've seen them put on the floor.
Mrs. E:	Yes. They can have legs—a three-legged stool.
Remotivator:	And some have legs? You must have worked on a few, Mrs. G. You sound like you know quite a bit also, Mrs. E.
Mrs. E:	Oh, yes.
Mrs. G:	That's right, I did. I made curtain stretchers too.
Mrs. E:	There were two kinds of frames. There was a backing that went into the frame at the same time. Some

	made the material very stiff, till it was very, very . . . just so.
Remotivator:	Yes, I see. How many people could work on a quilt at one time?
	[*Many responses: "Two," "four," or "five."*]
Remotivator:	Mrs. C?
Mrs. A:	[*Laughs.*]
	I'd rather not.
	[*Laughs.*]
Remotivator:	You'd rather not work at all?
Mrs. A:	[*Laughs.*]
Remotivator:	Miss S, you said four or five?
Miss S:	Yes.
Remotivator:	Mrs. G?
Mrs. G:	I said four or five too.
Remotivator:	Mary?
Mrs. N:	To put it together?
Remotivator:	Yes. How many people can work on a quilt at one time do you think?
Mrs. N:	No more than two.
Remotivator:	No more than two. Anyone else? . . . How many people?
Miss M:	I haven't any idea.
Mrs. C:	About two or three, yeah.
Mrs. G:	It takes a couple to put the frame together.
Mrs. C:	Yeah. Put the frame together.
Remotivator:	Just to put the frame together? I see. And what has to be done next? . . .
Mrs. C:	With the frame?
Mrs. G:	Yes.
Remotivator:	Is the material tacked, or . . . ?
Mrs. E:	Seat three on both sides, and one on each end. They have different designs. They have a chalk, and they chalk the different designs . . . and the different threads.
Remotivator:	Sounds very well planned.
Mrs. E:	And it comes out pretty.

Remotivator:	What kinds of needles are used?
Mrs. G:	Darning ones.
Mrs. E:	Quilting needles. They'd be best. Yes.
Mrs. F:	A large needle.
Remotivator:	Are bone needles used or a steel needle?
Mrs. G:	No. It's a steel needle.
Remotivator:	And what special stitches are used?
Mrs. E:	Any special.
Mrs. G:	Sometimes a button hole stitch, sometimes a hemming stitch.
Remotivator:	Button hole or hemming stitches. Do you think . . . ?
Mrs. E:	A chain stitch or a cable stitch.
Remotivator:	Many different kinds. . . . Mrs. F, what did you say?
Mrs. F:	A running stitch.
Remotivator:	I see. . . . Was that all done by hand or by machine?
Mrs. E:	By hand.
Mrs. F:	By hand.
Remotivator:	How many pieces, or swatches, of material have to be cut?
Miss S:	According to the frame.
Mrs. C:	According to the size. . . .
Mrs. N:	Well, depends on the size.
Miss S:	All different sizes.
Remotivator:	According to the frame, Miss S?
Mrs. E:	According to the size of the bed.
Remotivator:	And according to the size of the bed. Fine.
Mrs. E:	You measure that.
Remotivator:	Measuring it first is important. . . . How long do you think it would take to make the quilt?
Mrs. G:	Months.
Miss S:	According to how many times you work on it.
Remotivator:	Certainly. The number of times you work on it. . . .
Mrs. G:	According to how many people are working on it.
Remotivator:	That's true. You said months.
Mrs. G:	Yes, because by the time the cotton is put in and the cover's made. . . .

Remotivator: It takes time. . . . Mary, what do you think?

Mrs. N: If you have a small one, it takes less time to put it together. A small quilt or a big one. . . .

Remotivator: Yes. It depends on the size. . . . Who has ever seen one made or helped to make one?

Mrs. G: I have.

Mrs. E: I did.

Remotivator: You've both had lots of experience.

Mrs. E: Always a patch quilt.

Mrs. G: I made it by patches, too.

Remotivator: Patchwork quilts mostly? Is there anyone else that helped to make one? Miss M . . . No? . . . You never did, Mrs. C? You must have, in Venezuela!

Mrs. C: They make it, but I didn't . . . I watch it. Little pieces and so. . . .

Remotivator: So you have seen them made . . . In what areas of the country do you think quilting is still done?

Mrs. G: In the West. That's where we sent ours after we got them done, to have them quilted.

Remotivator: You sent them out?

Mrs. G: Yes. We used to send them out there. Especially the patch quilts.

Remotivator: Especially patch quilts?

Mrs. G: They do wonderful work on them.

Remotivator: In what area of the country do you think quilting is still done?

Mrs. F: I think in the West.

Remotivator: In the West?

Miss S: I think any place.

Remotivator: I think that's true, perhaps in some farming areas of the country.

Mrs. E: They do it in Ireland yet.

Remotivator: Oh, they still do it in Ireland?

Mrs. E: They make the long thread, and
                                              [*Takes a long pause.*]
and save the material for it, and then they have both sides quilted so you can turn it any way.

Remotivator: Reversible?

Mrs. E: Yes.

Remotivator:	Tell me . . . if you ladies were invited to a quilting bee, what job would you prefer?
Mrs. C:	I watch!
Remotivator:	Oh!
Miss S:	I'd take the frame.
Remotivator:	You'd take the frame? Fine. What job would you like, Mrs. F, if you were invited to a quilting bee?
Mrs. F:	Sew the patches together.
Remotivator:	Good. You'd sew the patches together. . . . Mrs. E, if you were invited to a quilting bee, what job would you like?
Mrs. E:	Patches are not so good, 'cause they're all going to do something of that, no matter what part they'd be working on, and I'd be nervous about how it was all getting together, so it wouldn't be useless.
Remotivator:	The putting it together; you would like fitting it into the chalked design?
Mrs. E:	Yes. It is very interesting.
Remotivator:	Mrs. W, if you were invited to a quilting bee, what part of the work would you like to do?
Mrs. W:	I don't know.
Remotivator:	You wouldn't know?
Mrs. W:	I don't know anything about the making of a quilt.
Remotivator:	But you said you'd like to do sewing.
Mrs. W:	If that job is vacant, but there's lots of others, like myself, you know.
	[*Laughs.*]
Remotivator:	Well, if you were the first one there, maybe you'd get the plain sewing part of it.
Mrs. E:	I think the hemming is very interesting too.
Remotivator:	The hemming?
Mrs. E:	The hemming and knotting them together. Many times you'd change to different things at the party.
Remotivator:	And do a little of each part of the work?
Mrs. E:	Yes.
Remotivator:	Mrs. A, would you like to work on sewing a quilt?
Mrs. A:	No. No . . .

Remotivator:	That doesn't interest you? There are other things you might like to do?
Mrs. A:	[*Laughs.*]
Remotivator:	Mrs. T, what part would you like, if you were invited?
Mrs. T:	Mm-mm-mm. Maybe crochet.
Remotivator:	You would just want to crochet one?
Mrs. T:	Mm-mm-mm. Maybe.
Remotivator:	That's good, I'll take the one you crochet!
	. . . [*Laughter.*]
	Miss M?
Miss M:	Make the design.
Remotivator:	You like to arrange the designs for the quilt, that's nice. . . . And Mary?
Mrs. N:	I'm making one now, so gotta make first the patches, and then put them together.
Remotivator:	Yes. What part would you like to do if you were invited? What would you like to do best?
Miss N:	The patches.
Remotivator:	Well, that's good. I hope we get a nice quilt out of that!
	[*Laughter.*]
Mrs. E:	When I first came to this country, I brought some warm quilting.
Remotivator:	You brought some from the old country?
Mrs. E:	Coming out here in 1906, I brought them from my aunt.
Remotivator:	That's nice. Do you still have any of them that you worked on?
Mrs. E:	Ah, no, I haven't. Right now, I haven't any.
Remotivator:	Your daughter doesn't have any?
Mrs. E:	I have a patch quilt I made since. I have a very nice one. Specially cut and shaped.
Remotivator:	Oh, I'm sorry, I didn't know. If I had known, I would have asked you, or had your daughter bring it in, so we could have shown it.
Mrs. E:	Sure, that's all right.

Remotivator:	Well, I have really heard a great many things about quilts I never knew. So much work and thought has to go into handmade quilts. I guess that's why they are so beautiful and so prized. I enjoyed talking about quilts with all of you today. Okay, Mrs. E, thank you for coming to the meeting today. You were very interesting.
Mrs. E:	T'was very nice.
Remotivator:	Mrs. W, next time we'll talk about dresses. I think you will enjoy that more.
Mrs. W:	[*Laughs.*] That's for another time.
Remotivator:	Mrs. A, thank you for coming this morning. I hope you enjoyed it.
Mrs. A:	[*Laughs.*]
Remotivator:	Mrs. T, thank you for coming to the meeting.
Mrs. T:	[*Smiles and shakes head.*]
Remotivator:	We should have had your daughter bring in the quilt you crocheted.
Mrs. T:	Mmm-mm-mm.
Remotivator:	Maybe she can bring it in another time.
Mrs. T:	No. She's away.
Remotivator:	She's on vacation? When she comes back. Mrs. C, thank you for coming to the meeting.
Mrs. C:	Yeah. I like.
Remotivator:	Miss M, thank you for coming and for reading the poem. It was very nice. We all enjoyed it.
Remotivator:	Mary, thank you so much for coming. I'll be looking forward to seeing your quilt when it's finished.
Mrs. N:	My pleasure.
Remotivator:	Mrs. G, thank you for coming, and for all the information you gave.
Mrs. G:	Okay.
Remotivator:	Thank you. . . .
Miss S:	Maybe we'll make a quilt now! [*Laughs.*]
Remotivator:	Okay, we'll do that. Mrs. G, want to make a quilt?
Mrs. G:	Yes.

Remotivator: Fine.

    Miss S: When you have the time. . . .

Remotivator: Mrs. F, thank you. It was a pleasure to have you here. . . . We'll plan to meet next Wednesday at ten o'clock, since I'm off next Tuesday. Okay? . . . and maybe we'll talk about dresses and fashions. How about that?

                                    [Affirmative response from several.]

In the meantime, I can speak to Sister in O. T. upstairs, and she can help those who want to work on quilts. Okay? See you next Wednesday.

Questions and Answers about Remotivation Therapy

Is remotivation a form of psychotherapy?   No. Remotivation usually deals with noncontroversial topics, topics that are objective instead of subjective. The discussions center around realities of everyday life and use topics like holidays, nature, fashion, current events, birds, hats, food, history, etc. The technique focuses on the "unwounded" areas of the personality, leaving the "wounded" areas for psychotherapists to deal with.

Even if we deal with objective topics, would not some of the topics involve sensitive areas and feelings?   Yes, but the remotivator, generally not a trained psychotherapist, accepts what is said by the patient without exploring the feelings. For example, at one session where Christmas was being discussed, one woman began to cry. She told the group that her husband had died on Christmas Day. The remotivator expressed her sorrow over the woman's loss and then continued the session which was on Christmas foods. The woman stopped crying and joined in the discussion, focusing on the special foods she had cooked that her husband had enjoyed. A trained psychotherapist may be asked to see this patient later in order to explore the feelings she expressed during the remotivation session.

What topics would not be used in remotivation sessions?   In general, topics like death, religion, love, sex, and politics would not be used. It has been found, however, that in some facilities aged individuals have had stimulating discussions on controversial topics like the generation gap, politics, remarriage, etc. The remotivator should use his sensitivity in deciding if his particular group would benefit from discussions dealing with more controversial topics.

If it is just a discussion group, why is it a special technique?   Because it is designed to meet the special needs of those who need more stimulation to promote interaction with others. Thus, the technique places the remotivator physically in the center of the group where he can move about freely to lead or dominate the action by providing extra stimulation. There is a definite framework that the remotivator uses in order to develop the discussion topic. Moreover, the technique focuses on just one topic instead of several. The discussion group does not meet to socialize. In summary, remotivation therapy is a structured, primarily leader-dominated discussion technique that explores an objective topic.

Are compliments important? Can't the group members interpret them as being false and insincere?   Compliments are a form of reinforcement through which specific behaviors are encouraged. Instead of being insincere, the remotivator uses positive comments with which he is comfortable. For example, remotivators have found that calling attention to the way a particular resident's hair may look after a trip to the beauty parlor or commenting on an attractive dress someone is wearing are often statements received with pleasure. Each remotivator should take special care to include each person so that no one person will feel neglected. Compliments may also include some factual information that the individual would like to share, such as the fact that "Mrs. N has just become a great-grandparent." The remotivator who knows his residents uses such available knowledge in the meeting as a way of enhancing this total *climate of acceptance.*

If we include a couple of confused residents in the group, don't we run into objections by the other group members?   That may happen. If the behavior of the more confused person leads to rejection by the others, plans should be made to redesign the group and place the confused person elsewhere. If the person's behavior is disruptive and if the remotivator's attempts to focus the patient's attention are not effective, the remotivator may have to remove the person from the group for the remainder of that session. It has been found that group members will often act in a protective way, trying to explain to the confused person what is being said, giving the person the "right answer," etc. If this happens, one of the direct goals of remotivation is being met, i.e., that of stimulating interaction among group members.

During one particular session the authors observed a confused resident stand up and move her chair back as though to walk away. The remotivator stopped and said, "I hope you can stay with us, Mrs. B." But the resident said no and wandered out of the room. The discussion continued and a short time later the resident returned and sat down again. The remotivator commented, "I'm so glad to have you back, Mrs. B. You were missed." The remotivator then continued as though nothing had happened. Residents should not be forced to attend remotivation sessions. Instead, they should be encouraged and invited to come back again.

Do remotivation sessions always start with questions?
Sometimes the remotivator can use a poem that leads into the topic. This is actually the way remotivation began, by reading poetry and asking questions. For example, "Trees" by Joyce Kilmer could lead into the topic of beauty. Sometimes a newspaper item or a quotation could be used, but this depends on the level of the group.

Does it matter what kind of poetry is used? Yes. The poem should be simple, objective, and appropriate to the topic. The poem should be rhythmic and it should rhyme. If it is well read, poetry is generally received with pleasure. Residents often applaud at the end to indicate their pleasure. Gloomy, depressing poems or poems that are difficult to understand should not be used.

What do you do when you cannot find a poem that fits the topic? One way would be to start with a related poem that could lead into the topic. Another way would be to use a poem that mentions the topic. Still another way would be to write your own poetry.

Are there other ways of giving rewards besides using compliments? Yes. Other forms include using one's smile, having a "warm" facial expression, and using eye contact. In addition, verbal reinforcements like "yes," "that's true," "fine" are also rewards and encourage further contributions from the group members.

What do you do if someone in the group gives a wrong answer? An honest feedback should be given for incorrect information. If the remotivator feels that the group member did not hear the question, he may simply rephrase or repeat the question. If the response is still incorrect, the correct one is provided by saying, for example, "Easter is a spring holiday," or by asking another group member and trying in that way to elicit a correct answer from him.

Does the remotivator need to know a lot about the topic being used? He does not need to be an expert, but he is expected to review basic information before the session starts.

Where could one find the information one needs for a remotivation session? Good sources of information are newspaper articles, magazine clippings, stories and pictures about such famous people as inventors, soldiers, painters, movie stars, and articles on soap making, stamp collecting, printing, television shows, movies, etc. Co-workers and other remotivators are also good resources. Library materials such as encyclopedias and dictionaries may also be consulted.

Where does the remotivator get all the props he needs for a session? Props may be obtained from departments in the remotivator's own facility, for example, the recreational therapy department, the occupational therapy department, and the dietary department. The remotivator may also use items that he or other people have collected.

Do the residents ask questions during the meeting? Yes. Usually the remotivator throws the question out to the group first. It has been found that someone usually comes up with an answer, but if no one does, the remotivator supplies the answer. If a group member asks a question that no one, including the remotivator, can answer, the remotivator may say, "Mrs. S had a very good question. Since none of us knows the answer, perhaps we can look it up later and let everyone know." The promise, once made, is always kept and the information, once collected, is shared with the group.

Does the remotivator ever have a session in which the group does not respond? That seldom happens. However, where individuals do not respond spontaneously, the remotivator should direct a specific question to one of the residents, for example, "Mrs. S, what other things could people do to celebrate July 4th besides watch a parade?" Many times a withdrawn resident participates just by remaining in a group and observing and listening to what is happening around him. This is accepted, but he should be encouraged to participate more fully.

Do the residents ever get into arguments in the session? Yes. Some residents interact by being argumentative. When the remotivator sees difficulties occurring that tend to foster disruption in the group, he can intervene just as he does when the group strays from the topic or when an overly talkative resident monopolizes the session. For example, he can introduce a summarizing comment and then redirect the group's attention to the next idea.

Do the residents enjoy the session? Remotivators have stated that residents genuinely enjoy the sessions. It has been observed that they talk about a session for days after it has taken place with other residents, staff, family members, and visitors.

Can the remotivator offer his own comments in a session? It is very important for the remotivator to feel that he is part of the group and it has been found that the remotivator who adds comments of his own often enhances the interaction of the group. However, this does not mean using his leadership role to monopolize the conversation. He should interact but he should not take over.

How do remotivators feel about the technique? It has been found that, in general, remotivators have expressed deep feelings of satisfaction and personal reward from their experiences leading remotivation sessions. They have reported that the information they learned from the residents during a session helped them understand these residents as individuals who have varied backgrounds and experiences. Remotivators have also reported that they were not aware that they could be group leaders and were delighted to find that they could be effective group leaders to whom others responded. They stated that the technique enhanced their own feelings of self-esteem and self-satisfaction.

Charting Progress

In order to keep an accurate record of the patient's progress, the patient's behavior should be charted after each remotivation session (see Appendix D). In this way the remotivator can observe the effects of the session on the patient's behavior, i.e., the interaction of the patient while in the group setting. Accurate records maintained over several months will indicate how well the patient is progressing in the group.

On the remotivation evaluation form the remotivator checks that number which corresponds most closely to the patient's response to the task described during *that particular session only*. For example, if the patient seemed to usually participate in the remotivation session, the remotivator would check "2" as the appropriate rating for the patient during that session. If, however, the patient seemed to participate "sometimes" during that session, then his rating would be "1." The patient's level of enjoyment would be rated in the same way. The form is filled out in *triplicate,* one for the medical chart (placed there at the end of a month), one for the remotivator, and one for the remotivator's supervisor.

In order to determine the general effect of the remotivation program, the remotivator might ask other staff personnel if they have noticed any different kinds of behavior in the patient since he started remotivation or since the last few sessions, etc. The remotivator then could use this information in subsequent sessions. For example, if the patient had not been generally helpful to others and now appears to be helpful, the remotivator might enlist his aid in helping other patients, for example, he could help move wheelchair patients. A consistent scoring of "2" ("usually") would indicate that the patient could be ready for a higher level of group, e.g., discussion, group therapy, art therapy, etc.

9

implementation of the step-ladder approach

Overall Goals

No matter what the modality, the primary goal is to keep every patient functioning at his optimal level. Since all patients are individuals and, therefore, at a variety of levels, there is a possibility for a wide range of goals. For example, the patient who is acutely ill with a stroke may seem to respond as his confusion lifts and he may eventually be rehabilitated to his own home, but the frail elderly person who has long-standing chronic brain syndrome may show confusion that will never decrease. For the former, there will be promotion from one modality to another, e.g., from sensory training to reality orientation to remotivation, etc., and perhaps eventual return to the community. Most likely the latter will be maintained for an extended period of time in a sensory or a reality group.

Basic to all of the modalities is the goal of increasing interpersonal skills and the number and quality of interactions. For the most regressed patients, this may mean 'only' the establishment of eye contact after many seemingly nonproductive sessions. For others, there may be a rapid improvement in grooming habits as a result of group participation. For some, there may be an incentive for independence in the activities of daily living (ADL), e.g., if a resident wants to get to his group meeting, he will be more attentive to dressing himself. Certain residents will become more cognizant of others' needs, e.g., in time one resident may choose to wheel a wheelchair-bound roommate to the sessions. All of the above may be instrumental in maintaining or possibly raising self-esteem and in minimizing apathy, withdrawal and, hopefully, even depression.

It must be remembered that for the residents involved, rehabilitation potentials and goals are often *limited*. Nevertheless, one must remember how even little successes can improve the quality of life in the closed environment of the institution. In addition, programs may appear childlike, but be rehabilitative in nature.

Matching the Group Leader
to the Technique

Not only do patients vary in that each patient should be assigned a particular therapeutic modality based upon the team's estimation of his need, but each group leader or therapeutic agent also varies in personal style and preference. Since sensory training is a technique that requires a great deal of touch contact with the patient, it has been found most helpful to recruit staff who can touch the patient easily. If the group leader cannot touch patients without feeling uncomfortable, he should be encouraged to lead one of the other techniques such as reality orientation therapy or remotivation. Reality orientation is a technique that emphasizes an approach that is mostly verbal. The remotivation technique is most akin to a formal classroom structure. It has been found that leaders who have difficulty with sensory training because they do not like to touch the patients do very well in a technique like remotivation therapy that does not require close contact with the patients. Every technique requires that the leader and the group establish rapport and that the leader like what he is doing and be empathic toward his group members. Therefore, the group leader should, whenever possible, choose the technique he is most comfortable with so that both the patients and the leader benefit the most from this endeavor. A way of determining which technique seems most "natural" is for the leader to try them all and choose the one that most suits his own style of relating to others.

The Team Approach

Most basic to all of the techniques is the *consistency* of the approach. Consistency can only be maintained if everyone who interacts with the resident is aware of what is going on with this person in terms of his level of functioning and assigned treatment approach. This is most easily done by using a team approach. That is, *everyone* who interacts with the resident, on any level, must be alerted to the fact that the patient is, for example, in a sensory training group and must be related to with that information in mind. This includes not only professional and paraprofessional ward personnel but others such as housekeeping and maintenance staff.

Team meetings should be held regularly and should include all staff who interact with the resident in order to inform them periodically of the resident's progress. The team should have a team leader who knows the residents well and who is able to maintain the team's cohesiveness. He should keep everyone informed of the patient's progress and he should have all the team members discuss problems and seek solutions to these problems. The team leader may be a nurse, social worker, activities worker, or perhaps an aide or an orderly.

It should be remembered that the various treatment programs outlined in this book are not to be perceived as limited programs occurring on a particular day for a limited period of time. Instead, they are to be considered as *approaches* to the resident. In other words, if a patient is in a sensory training or reality orientation group for a limited amount of time several times a week, the *approach* of sensory training should be an ongoing, 24-hour a day approach. This patient should be touched as often as possible and afforded as many opportunities as possible in order to develop his ability to discriminate stimuli. This approach should be used not only during group sessions but throughout the entire day by everyone who comes in contact with the patient. To be most consistent, staff persons from the recreation therapy and occupational therapy departments should also be made aware that this sensory training patient needs special attention paid to his inability to differentiate different textures, smells, tastes, etc.

Family Involvement

Members of the patient's family should be informed about the technique to which their aging family member has been assigned. The technique should be explained to them. They should be told that the technique is a total approach to be used by all persons who in any way interact with the patient. They should be asked to relate to the patient in a similar fashion and should be considered as adjunct staff. That is, if their family member is, for example, in a sensory training group, the rationale for this should be explained to them, the technique should be described, and they should be asked to use this approach in their interactions with the patient. They should be encouraged to touch the patient whenever possible and offer him various opportunities to develop his discriminatory capacities for different kinds of sensory experiences. For example, when the family member visits, he could offer the patient an orange and ask the patient how it tastes, if he likes it, or what it tastes like, i.e., is it sweet, very juicy, a little too tangy, etc. This could easily be included in normal conversation and it would prove very helpful to the total approach suggested. It has also been found that when family members are involved, their morale increases because they feel that something is being done for their aging family member and, most importantly, that they too are part of the therapeutic process. In addition, they are less prone to feeling that these techniques are too childlike. Family members are also informed of the patient's progress so that they are aware of how the patient is really functioning at different points in time.

The authors know of one family member, a wife, who was kept informed of her husband's progress in remotivation therapy. She also visited at different times while he was in session and was allowed to sit at some distance and observe him and the group (done with the patient's approval). After some time she offered to take her husband home. She explained that had she not observed her husband during remotivation sessions and seen behaviors she had no longer thought possible, she would never have concluded that he could function at home. She then took him home. Involving the wife in her husband's rehabilitation may have done much to restimulate her interest in taking him home and uplifting her morale to the point that she felt that she could possibly care for him again in their home surroundings.

Relationship of Stimulation Techniques to Psychotherapy

Therapy may be conceived of as being that which is beneficial to others. Stimulation techniques may be considered a form of therapy, but they are not the same as psychotherapy. Psychotherapy is a form of treatment that is intrapsychic in nature. The patient's behaviors and current functioning are explored in terms of his past experiences and how they relate to the way he functions at the present time, e.g., what gets in the way of his functioning better. The therapist tries to give the patient some insight into his inner life and helps the patient to learn not to "trip over his own feet."

Stimulation techniques, although therapeutic in the broad sense, are not psychotherapy because the therapist, or group leader, does not explore the dynamics of the personality and he does not make any interpretations. Instead, he stays with the limited goals of each of the particular techniques he is using. In addition, where *cure* is often the goal of the individual who seeks psychotherapy, this is not the goal of stimulation techniques. The goal is that the patient be able to function on a higher level whenever possible, that is, go from a sensory training group to a reality orientation group, or, if this is not possible, stay in the original group but perhaps not regress further. The thinking here is that the stimulation of the group experience may retard or hold constant any natural regression that might take place more easily if there were no group exposure.

Some forms of psychotherapy, e.g., analytic, place much emphasis on *transference,* that is, the way in which the patient relates to the therapist as he once did to other significant figures earlier in his life, but this is not the focus of the stimulation techniques. Nevertheless, there is no doubt that every group member does relate to the group leader in a special way, i.e., the way in which he related to others in leadership positions. The group leader of these techniques does not, however, verbalize awareness in his interaction with the group. The group leader should make a mental note of the special way each group member relates to him and use this, as he does all information he gathers about each patient, for the patient's benefit. In other words, if a patient is particularly hostile toward the group leader, it is possible that some of the patient's early life experiences with important people in positions of authority were of such a negative nature for him that he reacts with hostility to others who are in that position of leadership today. The group leader should discuss this with the team. The team may then wish to suggest activities to increase the patient's sense of self-esteem; assign him to some leader-type roles or involve him in discussion groups. It must be remembered that the group leader should be *aware* of the patients' responses to him as *he* should be aware of *his* responses to each patient. This information should be shared with other team members.

Life Style and the Institution

In describing the preceding techniques we have focused on a group of institutionalized aged who have common characteristics, symptoms, and maladaptations, particularly in the interpersonal sphere. The most common characteristic was regression, although the degree of regression may vary. Similarly, there was variation in the amount of social interaction. Thus, patients were categorized and matched to a technique best suited to their level of functioning.

There are, however, other forms of activity that may also be therapeutic for the patient residing within an institution. In order to be able to best match the activity to the patient, a thorough understanding of the patient's lifelong style of functioning is critical.

Although there is a tendency to label all adults over the age of 65 as "aged" or "aging," each of these persons is, in actuality, a unique individual, continuing in his older years the life style that was his when he was younger. The term *life style* itself, coined by Alfred Adler, is defined as "one's characteristic pattern of movement. . . . It includes a unique method of perceiving, conceptualizing, behaving, and striving toward a subjectively determined goal."[1] Each individual, then, is different from all others. Since there is a continuity of personality structure, the professional who works with the aging adult cannot view the patient in terms of his current situation only; instead, the person's way of interacting with his environment is a reflection of his past ways of coping, i.e., behaviors he has learned throughout his life. The whole person is also more than the sum of his parts. Therefore, he cannot be explained by focusing on a part of him such as the current disability, e.g., CVA, diabetes, etc. Although the current disability does influence the person in his social, emotional, and physical ways of coping, the total person determines the meaning this current ailment has to him.

Personnel who work with the aging individual must have some awareness of the particular life style of that person. This gives them clues to the person's pattern of movement such as the ways in which he perceives, thinks, feels, and acts toward the environment. Included are his particular biases, unique points of view, special

---

[1]J. W. Croake, "An Adlerian View of Life Style," *Journal of Clinical Psychology* **31** (1975): 513–518.

"colored glasses" he uses for perceiving and interpreting events around him, etc. Thus, there are cues to be picked up from the aging patient. To illustrate this concept of picking up on cues from the patient, let us look at a situation that was observed in a nursing home. Many patients were sitting around, involved in what may be termed the *doing nothing* syndrome, i.e., staring off into space while sitting in their wheelchairs or vacuously watching the blaring TV as they sat somewhat near each other (but in no way involved) on benches along the side of the large dayroom or in front of the TV. Suddenly an aging female patient, dressed similarly to the others (housedress with slippers), came into the room. As she deftly manipulated her walker along the floor, she called out orders to the other patients in a strident, dominant voice, "You there—move over there. You, I told you to sit in that other chair before, so get into it. You now—push your wheelchair closer to her," etc. A staff member soon came in and brusquely ordered her out of the dayroom. Cursing and mumbling to herself, the patient was eased out by the staff member.

Although this patient's behavior was aggressive, it suggested that this person had some sense of order and a need to control by "doing something" that would permit her to exercise this control. Instead of whisking her out of the room, the staff member should have recognized the need underlying the overt behavior and should have catered to it by moving the behavior in a positive direction. This patient could have been used to, perhaps, sort laundry or organize the seating arrangements of an anticipated bingo game, movie night, or birthday party. In other words, her need to organize, manipulate, and control others should have been diverted toward a positive way of behaving that would have benefited other patients, staff and, most importantly, herself. When this was not done, it should have been anticipated that this patient's behavior would continue, to no one's benefit and everyone's detriment.

10

additional therapeutic approaches

Activities Therapy (Recreation Therapy)

Another way of dealing with individual behaviors in the institutional setting and helping the patient function at his maximum potential is through activities therapy.[1] Paul Haun, one of the authorities writing on recreation states that recreation is a "primary need of all people."[2] Other authors have consistently stated that recreational activity adds greatly to the general "physical and mental vigor of the resident."[3] Most often, the aging person himself is not involved in seeking out a recreational activity he would like to pursue. More often than not activities are imposed by the administration and the choices are either minimal or nonexistent. This stripping away of choice mitigates against the fostering of continuity with his former life style. Avedon suggests that

> . . . recreation is generated from within oneself—another person may act as a catalyst, a specific object or act may have an attracting valence quality, but no force outside the self can make a person experience recreation.[4]

[1]H. D. Meyer and C. K. Brightbill, *Community Recreation: A Guide to Its Organization,* 3rd ed. (Englewood Cliffs, N.J.: Prentice-Hall, Inc., 1964).

[2]P. Haun, *Recreation: A Medical Viewpoint* (New York: Bureau of Publications, Teachers College, Columbia University, 1965), p. 39.

[3]W. Donahue, "Restoration and Preservation of Personality," in *Geriatric Institutional Management,* eds., M. Leeds and H. Shore (New York: G. P. Putnam's Sons, 1964), p. 180.

[4]E. M. Avedon, "Aging, Apprehension and Apathy," in *Recreation: Issues and Perspectives,* eds., H. Brantley and H. D. Sessoms (Columbia, S.C.: Wing Publications, Inc., 1969), p. 89

Thus, recreation should be one of the areas within the institution where the patient has a choice. He may choose, first, whether he *wants* to participate in any activities at all, and second, *which* activities he will attend. Recreation functions, in the institution as in the community, as a way of improving the quality of life.

Using this as a theoretical underpinning for recreational service, the worker must understand the different types of personality so that he can "fit" the personality to the activity. The person who is now a resident of an institution but who never played cards and has no desire to do so cannot be pressured into playing cards. The resident who was not socially gregarious in earlier years is not likely to become so now, particularly in the institutional setting.

Rehabilitative settings that are truly rehabilitative in nature work toward this goal of allowing and fostering independence in the resident. Recreation, a means of achieving this goal, must be designed to offer the widest range and variety of opportunities for the resident. He must be encouraged not only to make choices but also decisions that would affect him. Recreation should be a way of both strengthening the resident's contact with reality and encouraging the use of his particular abilities and skills. In this way, the resident is involved in creating his own human environment. It is easy for the professional to check off the persons he wants to attend a particular recreative function as a way of pleasing his supervisor, official investigators, etc., but a more beneficial way of functioning is for the professional to *ask* the resident what his preferences are.

planning an activities program

In planning any program of activities, it is necessary to remember the essential ingredient: the individual personality of the aging person. One can say that leisure activity is an aspect of personality. In studies it has been found that there was remarkably little change in *choice* of leisure activity as related to age (ages chosen ranged from 40 to 70 years). It was found that the significance of the leisure activity was more closely related to personality than to age, sex, or social class.[5] The amount and style of an aged person's participation are extensions of the patterns begun in childhood and shaped in adulthood. For example,

---

[5]R. J. Havighurst, "The Leisure Activities of the Middle Aged," *American Journal of Sociology* **63** (1957): 152–162.

persons active throughout the life span will retain this style in their later years although activity levels may be modified by alterations in life situations such as physical limitations. For example, the older person may find himself slower and less agile and thus may find himself unable to continue to play 18 holes of golf—9 may suffice or just teeing off on a lawn may be realistic. When even this is impossible, he may have to be content to watch golf matches on television. The point is that a person generally does not become active or sedentary in later life; instead, he *continues* doing what he has done *all of his life.*

recreation activities

Below is a list of the recreation activities that are often included in activities programs at various facilities. It is in no way a complete list and is intended to be a guide. The important factor to remember is that there should be activities offered from all of the following categories:

1. *Individual activities*
   Crossword puzzles (large print if available)
   Jigsaw puzzles
   Reading
   Television viewing
   Creative writing
   Visiting with relatives, friends, or volunteers
   Photography
   Knitting
   Crocheting
   Sewing
   Painting
   Crafts
2. *Small group activities*
   Current events discussion
   Documentary movies
   Dramatics
   Body movement
   Music appreciation group
   Men's and women's club
   Bible discussion
   Poetry group
   Political action group

Gourmet club
Sensory training
Reality orientation
Remotivation
Group therapy
Residents council
Crafts
Choral group
"Around the world" club
Trips
Cards and games
Dance and art therapy

3. *Large group activities*
Feature films
Garden parties
Wine and cheese parties
Picnics
Cocktail parties
Trips
Birthday parties
Bingo
Holiday celebrations
Entertainment

4. *Religious activities*
Services—regularly scheduled services, e.g., Protestant, Catholic, Jewish
Clergy visits
Holiday observances
Ethnic celebrations

Individual activities. Individual activities are engaged in by all residents whether formally or informally. Many residents may obtain reading and handiwork material from family and friends, but for others obtaining these items may serve as the first step in establishing rapport between the resident and the activities staff. The possibilities for activities are, of course, unlimited and the worker must be guided by the residents' skills and interests. Volunteers can be most effective in introducing and guiding individual activities.

When the institutionalized resident is sitting alone, he is often pushed to join an activity. It has been suggested, however, that there is a need for some aged people to have opportunities to develop the art of aloneness.[6] Being alone can be enjoyable if it is a *voluntary* aloneness. The person who works with the aged must decide, again by observing behavior and by talking with the patient, whether the need to be alone is a life style that is to be respected or whether the patient feels lonely and wishes to become involved. If the latter is the case, the worker should be there to help him with that task.

Small group activities. Small group activities should be developed when there are several residents who have similar interests, e.g., a dramatics club, a choral group, a poetry-reading group, or regularly scheduled offerings that may not necessarily attract the same residents each time, e.g., documentary films, current events, discussions, and trips. Small group activities are the core of a well-planned activities program because they necessitate active involvement on the part of the resident. Involvement and interest mitigate against apathy, withdrawal, and possibly depression. The number and type of these activities will vary from time to time according to the interests, education, and skills of the resident population as well as the availability of appropriate activity leaders. Special interest groups may be led by interested and capable residents or volunteers as well as activities leaders or other staff. For example, in a facility in which the activities staff is all female, the men's club may be led by a male administrator or other staff member. In addition, a language class may be conducted by a bilingual resident. An interested nurse may wish to lead a "Keep Well Club," or the chef may guide the "Gourmet Club." Moreover, small groups may be created to accommodate the interest of community groups. For example, if members of the local women's club wish to present a few sessions on flower arranging, this can be easily integrated into the schedule.

A few words of caution: There may be some residents who may participate only in small groups or only in a few individual activities. They may be reluctant to mingle in crowds because they may feel that they do not "fit in" with everyone or because they may have very specific interests and needs. This has probably been a lifelong pattern for them and their response represents a continuity of life style. This life style is to be respected.

---

[6]I. F. Ehrlich, "Lifestyles among Persons 70 Years and Older in Age-Segregated Housing," *The Gerontologist* **12** (1972): 27–31.

Large group activities. Large group activities generally require the least amount of interaction. For this reason, we might suggest that they are sometimes the least therapeutic. Paradoxically, they are the most frequent forms of activity because they present the best image of the facility to visitors. In addition, they often require the least amount of professional input, e.g., one person can run a film for 150 residents or one caller can call "Bingo" for a roomful of people. Nonetheless, large group activities are useful and necessary as long as they are not the *only* available activities. In reality, people in the community play "Bingo" and go to the movies when they wish, but they also engage in other activities. Thus, the same choices should be made available to the residents in a facility.

Large group programs may be made exciting and special, e.g., monthly birthday parties or entertainment by celebrities may encourage residents to "dress up" and prepare for a major event. In addition, they may provide a very pleasant means of attracting families to visit with the residents. Also, the value of the use of community people to provide entertainment must not be underestimated because it is most important that residents maintain a link with the outside world. Among the most common large group activities are birthday parties, special holiday meals, entertaining films, musical programs, and (you guessed it) "Bingo."

Religious activities. Although it is debatable whether or not religious interest increases as one gets older, religious activities must be provided not only because of Medicare and Medicaid regulations but also because, again, there must be a continuity of life style.[7] Regular religious services should be offered and clergy should be encouraged to make individual visits on a regular basis. In some facilities residents may wish to assist with services or even conduct them. For example, in one facility a resident played the organ for the Protestant services. The kind and scope of religious activities should be governed by the resident population. Thus, there would probably be daily services in a church-sponsored facility and weekly services in a nonsectarian facility. Moreover, scheduling should be governed by space limitations and other

[7]D. Blazer and E. Palmore, "Religion and Aging in a Longitudinal Panel," *The Gerontologist* **16** (1976): 82–85.

institutional realities. Regardless of the setting, interested patients should be encouraged to practice their beliefs and rituals as they wish, both formally and informally.

goals of activity therapy

Generally, a good activities program improves the quality of life within a facility. As stated previously, activities help the patient function at his optimum level and thus foster independence, a sense of identity and purpose, and the opportunity to *make choices*. A program is therapeutic if it helps the patient toward these goals. Realistically, many of the activities are diversionary, but recreation is, and should be, primarily *fun*. Recreation is about the only service in a facility that cannot be precisely prescribed. Thus, although current legislation requires physicians to order activities for the residents, no one can say, "Give this patient 2 gm of recreation." But a physician could order that "increased socialization" be encouraged. The method by which these orders are implemented should be devised by the recreation therapist and his staff.

criteria for success

The success of a program in institutional settings is too often measured in terms of the numbers attending. Although some indications of success may sometimes be measured in terms of the numbers attending, this indicator seems inadequate. This is true even in community settings where it may be assumed that an individual has more choice. That is, camp programs for aging persons in the community may also be measured this way, i.e., the recreation hall program is considered a failure or success that night strictly by a *count* of persons, not by the *meaning* of the experience to the people attending.

The general atmosphere of the home and the morale of the residents may be more effective measures for judging the success of programs. Persuading residents to participate in programs not to their liking also adds to issues of persuasibility and authoritarianism.[8] This relates to the point of whether or not participation by the residents is a reflection of their exercising

---

[8]R. G. Bennett, "The Meaning of Institutional Life," *The Gerontologist* **3** (1963): 64.

options, i.e., is the program offering them opportunities for a meaningful experience? Observation of such factors as interest, involvement, frequency of participation, enjoyment, growth, and socialization would provide clues for assessing this.

time and frequency

Activities should be available during as many of the working hours as possible *every day* of the week. That residents "want" to go to bed early is a myth and generally reflects the fact that there is nothing for them to do in the evenings. Similarly, the often-heard statement that there should not be activities during visiting hours is indicative of the staff's attitudes instead of the residents' wishes. Obviously scheduling activities must take institutional realities into account. For example, activities should not be scheduled until enough time has elapsed after breakfast for morning care, medications, etc., to be taken care of. Moreover, activities should not be scheduled in a room that is being used for other purposes, such as team conferences or in-service programs. It may be desirable, however, to schedule an activity during a mealtime, e.g., a picnic or an ethnic celebration. Conflicts with other therapies, such as physical therapy or speech therapy, are generally best resolved between patient and therapists. Thus, if a patient likes "current events" and it is only scheduled at 10:00 a.m., perhaps the physical therapist could schedule him at another time that day. Ideally, each staff member should be aware of a patient's complete daily schedule through some sort of charting device.

How much or how often a resident participates is highly individual and depends to a great extent on the resident's interest and motivation. If the resident appears to be apathetic and if the professional feels that a particular activity may be "good" for the patient, there might be a temptation for the professional to push him into that activity without asking him whether or not he would enjoy the activity. Here, the professional is acting in an authoritarian way and it may be questioned how beneficial that activity will be to the patient. It is often asked whether gentle coaxing is helpful if the team or the professional worker strongly feels that the patient needs the recreation being offered. This is a difficult question to answer. The answer must come from the team and there should be maximum input from the patient whenever possible. However, *coaxing* is different from *pushing!*

a written schedule

A written schedule of activities should be prepared either on a weekly or monthly basis. A few large, attractive poster-sized schedules should be prepared for posting on bulletin boards and in other strategic places, e.g., in the dining room or the front lobby. In addition, individual copies of the schedule should be distributed to each resident and to administration and other department heads. If the program is extensive and if the budget and staff warrant it, monthly program booklets may be prepared. The activities worker may post the individual schedules in a strategic place, e.g., near the mirror or on the closet door, for slightly confused residents. Although the schedules should be attractive, they should be uncomplicated and very legible. It is also suggested that annotated schedules be sent to other department heads with requests for assistance, e.g., to dietary with a request for refreshments for the birthday party and the picnic.

the activities leader

Many facilities have only one staff member responsible for activities. In reality, this person more often serves as a coordinator than as an activities leader. He does *not* conduct every activity and, therefore, does not have to be a "jack of all trades." Instead, he is responsible for devising and implementing the activities schedule. Obviously, he must be familiar with the resources in the community. The more skillful he is in securing volunteer help, the more diversified his program will be. He must conduct many of the regularly scheduled programs such as the birthday party, the residents' council, cards and games tournaments, and various crafts programs. He should be warm, empathic, well-organized, flexible, and able to integrate and implement new ideas.

Today there is a tendency toward more regulation and professionalism. Larger facilities have a registered recreation therapist as director of activities and smaller facilities have a less trained person who works in conjunction with a qualified consultant who is a registered recreation therapist or a registered occupational therapist. Minimal training at this time varies from a designated course (ranging from 36 to 64 hours depending on the state) plus a specified period on the job, e.g., one year, to a master's degree program that involves not only course work but also supervised field experience. There is a trend toward certification by the National Therapeutic Recreation Society.

charting progress

The activities coordinator is responsible for keeping records on patient activities. Initially, he must put into the chart a record of an interview that reveals the patient's interests, hobbies, skills, and previous leisure experiences as well as expressed interest in the facility's activities. In addition, he must keep ongoing records of the patient's attendance and must put into each chart a monthly (or a quarterly) summary of progress. Progress notes should mention the patient's participation (or lack of it), changes in condition, successes or failures, and any modification of goals.

Of primary importance is the activities coordinator's ability to organize and transmit this information accurately and concisely. Since at this time there is no objective measure of activities programming, assessment depends on the activities leader's observations. Volunteers and co-leaders should be encouraged to report the patient's responses to the activities coordinator regularly. The activities coordinator, of course, should integrate this material into the chart notes.

Supportive Group Psychotherapy

The history of group therapy or *group* has shown rapid dramatic change. As recently as 25 years ago this approach was one of many for dealing with unhappy or unfulfilled people. It has since blossomed into a major social intervention, from traditional group therapy to the plethora of groups that exist today: encounter groups, human potential groups, sensitivity training groups, marathons, leaderless groups, etc.[9]

It has been found that in dealing with the aging individual the most suitable approaches are the supportive ones that emphasize resocialization of the person, a recognition of the need for promoting interdependence in the group, increased self-sufficiency, and increased potential for happiness. The traditional psychoanalytic group therapies attempt to deal with unconscious mechanisms such as motivations, defenses, fantasies, and resistances.

Despite the rapid advances of group, psychotherapy as a

---

[9]M. Rosenbaum and A. Snadowsky, *The Intensive Group Experience* (New York: The Free Press, 1976).

group experience involving older people has never been
readily available to the aged. Since therapy demands so much time
and effort, it is considered better to expend them on those who
have a long life ahead.[10] This may be partly a result of the influence
of Sigmund Freud who suggested that psychoanalytic treatment
was not particularly suitable for older people. Despite Freud's
pessimism, however, other analysts attempted to use
psychoanalytic approaches and reported positive effects.[11] Thus,
there has been a change in the use of therapy of this nature with the
older adult; the attitude that intervention with the aging person is
hopeless and that cure is almost impossible is undergoing a radical
change.

goals in supportive group approaches

The group approach may be viewed as a psychological process
in which a trained leader uses his particular skills to effect change
in persons selected for his group. Group therapy may be said to
have as its aim the promotion of better human relationships. For
the aging group member, modified goals of treatment may be
more realistic. Instead of focusing on personality reorganization, a
more supportive approach would be to offer guidance as a means
of catering to the patient's needs for assistance. In this approach
the patient's feelings of inferiority, acquired over a life span, are
met with reassurance and his anxiety is relieved by the therapist
who assumes a protective role. The patient's guilt is also relieved by
the therapist's permissive attitudes.[12]

A goal limitation is decided upon at the beginning of group
treatment. No attempts to reawaken old conflicts should be made
since it is assumed that each member's group style reflects a life
style that has been used to derive gratification for himself as a way
of protection against injuries to self-esteem. Defenses are thus not
tampered with. The therapist here is a relatively active person,
directing the course of therapy by providing guidance,
reassurance, and environmental manipulation whenever
necessary. He tries to decrease anxiety in the patient and promote a

---

[10]"The Old in the Country of the Young," *Time,* August 3, 1970, p. 50.

[11]M. Grotjahn, "Analytic Psychotherapy with the Elderly," *Psychoanalytic Review* **42** (1955): 419–427.

[12]A. I. Goldfarb, "Minor Maladjustments of the Aged," in *American Handbook of Psychiatry,* vol. 3, eds., S. Arieti and E. B. Brody (New York: Basic Books, 1974).

feeling of being understood. Further, and most important, the patient may be actively involved in solving his own problems. The therapist may also use some didactic measures, e.g., a discussion of what happens to the body as a result of aging, attitudes held by society toward the aging, ways of dealing with death, etc. The therapist and the patient should be involved in an intense, meaningful interpersonal relationship. Sometimes this is the *only* relationship in the patient's current life. Basically, supportive group therapy is a means of attempting to reestablish an emotional balance that has been shaken by the many stresses of later years, not the least of which has been a move from the community setting to the institutional one. Thus, even though the goals are limited, group therapy is known to have decreased the older person's fears and angers, improved his behavior and, in general, made for more optimal overall functioning.

target population

Theoretically, any patient who resides in a facility can be introduced to a group therapy program after some preparation. In actuality, however, because of the limited number of trained persons available, older persons selected for this approach are usually those who appear to be suffering from stresses with which they are unable to cope. For example, patients in one facility had to move from one floor to another. The authors observed that some patients seemed to manage very well but others seemed to "fall apart," i.e., they were more vulnerable. The latter patients should be assigned to group therapy so that they can be helped to deal with the current stress. Similarly, people who have difficulty getting along with others, people who appear very depressed, anxious, agitated or withdrawn, should also be assigned to group treatment.

composition of the group

Mixing personality types (heterogeneity) appears to benefit the group. Thus, a group may contain depressed patients, suspicious patients, "brain-damaged," or very regressed patients. If, for example, a group is made up of several depressed persons, it is often helpful to include some "starters" as part of the group, i.e., active, lively persons who act as catalytic agents to stimulate the entire group.

A group should generally consist of from 8 to 10 patients. If this is not feasible, there may be from 6 to 8. There should be enough group members to spur activity; if there are too few members, there will be many "dead" spots and there will be less spontaneity. Similarly, too many members will produce too much activity for both the leader and the group members. In addition, the more reticent patient may feel very lost in a large group.

Groups may be closed (the membership remains the same over a period of time) or open (the membership keeps changing). Once the group has been formed, other patients may ask to join. If possible, another group should be formed. If this is not possible, tact and patience should be used in explaining the exclusions. If it is possible that other groups will be formed in the future, the patient should be told this but *only* if this is a foreseeable reality. One should never raise false hopes.

time

Groups may meet for an hour and a half or two hours. However, it has been the authors' experience that groups of aging persons need less time. A group therapy session may last for an hour to an hour and a half without fatiguing its members. Sessions of less than an hour, e.g., 50 minutes, may also be helpful. The leader decides the time for the session because he knows the scheduled times of the other activities available to the patients during the day. The group therapy session should be scheduled at a time that is convenient to all.

frequency

The group may meet once or twice a week but it has been found that once a week is more practical because there is a shortage of trained personnel in this form of group therapy and because of the pressures of other duties and responsibilities these personnel have when they are available.

place

It is helpful to meet in a room that is attractive, well lit, and comfortable and where there will be as few disturbances as possible. The less distraction from the environment, the more energy can be devoted to the process taking place. In addition, the room should not be bare because a bare room makes for a depressing atmosphere and it should not be cluttered with objects because the clutter would be distracting.

Chairs should be arranged in a rough circle and there should be no table. The distance between chairs should be approximately less than one arm's length. If there were a table in the room and if patients were to sit around it, it would tend to dilute the process since members' bodies would be partially hidden from view. A seating arrangement in which everyone is easily seen is preferred. The therapist sits within the circle, preferably in a corner because the diagonal position offers the most advantage to observing all patients at all times.

materials

There are no special materials required for this group approach. It has sometimes been helpful to tape-record some of the sessions so that the group members can play them back for themselves. If the sessions are to be recorded, permission must be requested from the group for it has been found that some older persons are inhibited by the recording of the session. When permission has been sought and the goal explained, i.e., for teaching/helpful purposes, the recording of the session is often received with much enthusiasm by group members, many of whom have never had the opportunity to hear themselves on tape and are glad to have that chance now.

written schedule

A written schedule indicating the names of the persons in this program, the time, the place, the day, and the date of the meeting may be posted. More often than not, however, the schedule is not posted because, despite the advanced thinking of our time, there is still some stigma attached to the words "group therapy" and patients may not wish to have their names posted. Usually patients in a group therapy program are aware of all the details of the meeting and do not have to be reminded of it by having it publicly displayed. Again, the nature of the patients, the facility, and the reality requirements are to be the determining factors on this issue.

the leader

It is most important that the group therapy leader have adequate training in conducting groups. Along with this, personal qualities of intuitive insight, the ability to be empathic, and an in-depth understanding of himself are most helpful. He should not only be aware of himself, his own feelings, ideas, attitudes, and perceptions, he should also be aware of every group member and establish and maintain meaningful contact with each one. Since he plays a leading role, he should sometimes offer instructional information but he must be aware of when he is teaching too much. He should also have an optimistic attitude. When the group falters or seems unduly depressed, his optimism often is the most effective tool for rehabilitation. At times it may be difficult to maintain an optimistic attitude, but its value cannot be underestimated.

a therapy session: abbreviated notes of a recorded session (week eleven)

Below is an abbreviated example of a group therapy session conducted in a facility. The goal was to stimulate group interaction as a way of dealing with the members' expressed loneliness. In addition, support was given to the group members' attempts to find solutions themselves as a way of bolstering their egos. The therapist allowed herself to be seen as a guiding person who could help them accept dependency feelings and could encourage them to be independent. Memories from the past were encouraged as a way of integrating the past into the present life. These memories also provided clues to the therapist as to what resources the group member currently has. The resources were then supported as a further means of strengthening the person's ego, i.e., the ability to cope with the current reality. Similarly, the therapist discussed the "outside" world (Washington, D.C.) as a way of linking the patients' former lives to the current ones.

Mrs. R: It's good to be here for all reasons.

Therapist: What reasons?

Mrs. R: Well, because otherwise the week seems so long. It's a pleasure to come to talk to other people and to you, darling.

Mrs. C: That's it. When I stay in my room here too long, sometimes I talk to myself.

[*Laughs.*]

I talk to the walls too. Then I find something to do, like coming into the day room to watch TV. But how much TV can you watch?

Therapist:	How about the others?
Mrs. B:	We come here to be with everyone—you, the nurse, everyone.
Mrs. K:	How was Washington? Did you tell the president about us? [*Everyone laughs. Reference is to trip the group leader had recently made to Washington.*]
Therapist:	[*Spends a few minutes telling of trip to Washington and some sights visited.*]
Mrs. C:	Washington is where everything happens. They have to know to make things better for older people.
Mrs. K:	But 30 or 40 years ago we didn't even have this much. We just have to fight for things—then maybe you get some.
Therapist:	What kinds of things in particular were you thinking of?
Mrs. C:	Well, poor people have to be helped.
Therapist:	Could you spell that out—in what way?
Mrs. C:	Well, the poor are poor and the rich are rich. It could be better. But not only with money. Some people don't care for the poor people or the old people. It would take three hours to tell you. [*Sighs.*]
Therapist:	We don't have three hours but we have some time and I think maybe we can all discuss this. What do the rest of you think?
Mrs. C:	Mrs. R can tell you.
Mrs. R:	I can tell you that now it's better. We never had Social Security. Now we have that and they even send somebody to clean your house if you need it I am told. From this hospital they sent a girl three times a week to the man who used to live next door to me whose wife died. My daughter sees them and told me. They never used to do this.
Mrs. K:	If everybody pushes and fights, we'll get what we need.
Therapist:	Good point.
Mrs. B:	Believe me, we all worked all our lives and we should get things from this country.
Therapist:	Absolutely.

Mrs. K:	Will we be meeting some more?
Therapist:	How do you feel about that—do you want to?
Mrs. K:	Sure. This helps. Coming to the group is good.
Therapist:	In what way?
Mrs. K:	Well, in the group we talk to each other, see each other more.
Therapist:	You're saying you're lonely. What could you and all of us do about that?
Mrs. K:	We have to have more groups for us and even for some of the others, not just the one hour. That flies. The one hour is good but what is one hour? Last week Mrs. R (from another ward) came to sit in my room and talk to me for a while and it was a real pleasure.
Mrs. R:	[*Laughs.*]
	Then I invited her back. I wished I had some tea or something to give her but she said she just wanted my company.
Therapist:	I can understand that.
Mrs. H:	That's right. But we have to find things for us to do by ourselves—right, doctor? We have to keep busy—otherwise the day is so long.
Therapist:	Yes. A day can seem long if there is nothing to do. How about the rest of you—what do you think?
Mrs. C:	Right. We all have to help each other.
Mrs. K:	Back home—before here, I used to belong to clubs. That was the only thing that helped me—otherwise you think too much. It used to help pass the time when my son couldn't come to see me often—when he moved away. We even had a community center in the building and two evenings a week we used to go there and sing and tell stories. All the old people in the building used to go. It was nice.
Mrs. H:	We don't have a community center here—but we could get together by ourselves in the day room or someplace when the doctor is not here. We could just get together and talk to each other. The doctor said it was a good idea, right, doctor?
Therapist:	I think that's a fine idea. I would be glad to hear all

about it. Try it for next time and let's talk about it in the
group. See you next week.

[*States day and time.*]

So long until then.

questions and answers
about supportive group psychotherapy

What are the special qualities, if any, of the "good"
therapist? It has been said that the good therapist is an
astute observer, a thoughtful listener, a tireless collector of data, a
curious investigator, a disciplined clinician, and an independent
thinker.[13] Although this may define the ideal therapist, the
well-qualified therapist should have some combination of these
characteristics.

What happens when a group member dies? This
frequently happens in groups with the aged. When it does occur,
the death should be discussed. The therapist can bring it up by
saying something like, "I heard that Mrs. G died during the night,"
and wait for the group to respond. Exploration and in-depth
discussions of the death should be attempted. Discussion of the
death should not be avoided.

What if a group member says that he does not want to be in a
group with another group member? This sometimes happens.
Whenever possible, the suggestion should be made that it would be
helpful for him, Mr. A, to stay in the group because talking about
what bothers him about Mr. B could be very important to him and
to the others. If Mr. A still refuses, he should be gently told that the
group therapy sessions are voluntary and that he does not have to
remain. If it is possible, he should be placed in another group.

How about sex distribution in groups? Usually there are
many more females than males in the groups. If at all possible, a
more equal distribution should be attempted, but if this is not
feasible, it should help to have one or two men in a group with six
females. The group in which the sexes are mixed has a very
different quality from the group in which the members are the
same sex.

---

[13]K. Abraham, *Selected Papers* (London: Hogarth Press, 1948).

Doesn't talking about sex in a group containing older people in an institution raise problems about what to do about it? Yes, but sex and sexual activity are natural aspects of life and patients do have feelings about sex even though they do not talk about it. Discussing the subject in the group helps patients deal with these feelings. It is often an important area in which "life" can be brought back to the person. How to resolve the issue of sexual activity between partners in the institution can also be discussed and the group can be helped to find solutions to this problem.

When are the patients in a group "cured"? It all depends on the group and its members. Sometimes some members are ready to leave a group before others are ready to leave. At that point, new members may be brought into the group. The "cure" has to do with the goals of the group and the characteristics of the group and its members. There is no special time schedule for "cure."

Don't the other patients on the ward think of the person in group therapy as being crazy? That may be. The group therapy program can help the person in the group to deal with them and the slur.

Do the people in the group become closer to each other or more hostile? It depends on the person and the point of time in the group experience. Some people feel closer to others in the group, but some feel more hostile. These feelings should be discussed by the group. Often people in a group together become good friends on the ward and develop a closeness they had not shared before.

charting progress

Almost all group therapists keep records or progress reports of the sessions. Notes should not be taken during the session, but for the sake of accuracy, they should be written as soon after a session as possible. These notes are a way of keeping records of the group's progress and they indicate to the therapist the direction in which the group is moving. These records should be shared with other staff personnel because the records provide information about the person in the group that can greatly help staff in their planning activities with that patient. The group therapist should also make notes for himself about the particular behavior of a group member in order to alert other staff that, for example, Mr. A may be acting more depressed because of something he is going through in the group. This alerts ward personnel not to be punitive but to understand that the depression is being dealt with in the group and that it may decrease over time.

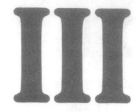

the
community
aged

11

the community aged

The vast majority of the aged do not live in institutions; they remain in the community. A significant proportion of this large group of older individuals remains very active, sometimes through participation in senior center activities. The community aged also become involved in church and other religious organization programs, remain employed as part-time workers, and are increasingly interested in continuing their education at various schools and colleges. Still others retain a strong family orientation by fulfilling grandparent and other roles.

Many of the community elderly can be observed sitting on benches in parks and other places where people gather. This 95 percent of the aged population is extremely varied, their needs and situations very individualized, and their problems and strengths very specific. The vast majority of this group might be called the *active aged,* in the sense that they comprise individuals who are physically healthy and fairly mobile. In contrast, the smaller proportion of the community aged might be termed the *passive aged,* in the sense that they are less ambulatory, perhaps in poorer health, but do not reside within an institution. The active aged comprise the majority of what is increasingly being termed the *young–old.* The young–old are people between the ages of 55 and 75 who are distinguished as a group by the common fact of having experienced retirement. According to the criteria, the young–old currently make up approximately 15 percent of the United States population. This age group is viewed by many social scientists as becoming ever more educated, being increasingly concerned with self-development, remaining psychologically and physically vigorous, and interested in discovering meaningful uses for their leisure time. It is expected that those who work with the community aged will be dealing more and more with the needs, hopes, and aspirations of such individuals. The passive aged will soon comprise the majority of what has recently been termed the *old–old*. The old–old, or those people 75 and over, may often continue to live in the community but become increasingly dependent on supportive social services and prosthetically designed physical environments. Although we have made some distinctions between the active aged and the passive aged and between the young–old and the old–old, we can still talk about some general problems faced by the community aged as a group.[1]

Problems of the Community Aged

The problems faced by the community aged might be described in terms of the following problem source areas: economic, physical, social, psychological, and philosophical. Each one of these source areas poses significant conflicts and stresses with which old people often have to cope. In fact, it is proposed that the goals of any comprehensive rehabilitation or service program could only be truly achieved by helping the elderly deal with all these problem source areas successfully. Unfortunately, most programs seem to focus on only a few of these source areas at any one time. Few programs seem to be equipped to assess and serve the full spectrum of needs. Below is an outline of these problem source areas and the stresses they induce.

Problem Source Area	*Related Stress*
Economic	Adjusting to income loss and to a new life style upon retirement.
Physical	Adjusting to the experience of body changes, some health deterioration, lowered mobility, and decreases in sensory capacities.
Social	Adjusting to potential loss of social status, no adequate replacement of social roles, and the need to evaluate leisure needs as independent of work.

---

[1]B. Neugarten, "Age Groups in American Society and the Rise of the Young Old," *Annals of the American Academy Political and Social Sciences* **415** (1974): 187–198.

Psychological	Adjusting to the realization of no longer being young and the resultant feelings about the self. New developmental tasks and crises become important, while old issues (such as *Who am I?*) reemerge and become newly central.
Philosophical	Coming to grips with existential and/or religious issues. The issues of *Why am I? What is my life about? What is life in general about?* come in to the foreground of thought.

Although people of all ages must deal with these issues, they are more salient as a group of problems for the aged. That is, the aged are often in the position of having to experience and cope with all of the above problems simultaneously. In contrast, younger persons usually have, at least momentarily, to resolve issues related to one or two of the above problem source areas and when stress experiences do occur, they are not as acute as they are for the aged.[2]

Tangible Approaches in the Counseling Mode

The methods and techniques of working with older people must inevitably differ from approaches used with younger people. In particular, counseling older people should focus on tangible interactions as opposed to purely interpersonal sensitivity group approaches. In other words, the counselor should use a topic, i.e., something tangible, as an environmental prop through which to relate. This general guideline has a number of advantages: First, it decreases anxiety among participants. Second, it creates a focus for counseling that is quickly understood by participants. Third, it provides options for the counselor, such as staying at content (superficial) information exchange levels versus going into personal (in-depth) feeling levels.

Something tangible is characterized by qualities that are immediately perceivable. Counseling approaches that might be characterized as tangible usually involve clear goals and purposes such as teaching skills, developing interests, or discussing topics. Structured, time-limited, problem-centered group approaches

---

[2]L. Gottesman, C. Quarterman, and G. Cohn, "Psychosocial Treatment of the Aged," in *The Psychology of Adult Development and Aging*, eds., C. Eisdorfer and M. Lawton (Washington, D.C.: American Psychological Association, 1973).

might be considered tangible because they provide external material through which individuals relate. Thus, the senior center that provides time for specific classes, training in specific skills, or discussion groups around specific topics might engender greater group and individual participation than a center that provides more abstract general counseling or therapy. This latter approach, although useful, might be more emotionally threatening or not as easily understood by members living in the community and is better reserved for those who specifically seek psychotherapy.

A number of group-based counseling intervention approaches have recently emerged that seem to deal with the problems engendered by the social, psychological, and philosophical problem source areas discussed above. One such approach, the *life enrichment counseling approach*,[3] and an approach that stresses *peer counseling*[4] will be presented below.

Life Enrichment

Any person's life history is a recording of his attempts to add positive experiences. Such experiences might be conceptualized as the "nutriments" necessary for an enriched life. It is only under certain conditions, such as increased stress, that this tendency toward life enrichment appears to wane, becomes inhibited, or is arrested. For example, the person who is forced to retire and whose main source of enrichment (nutriment) came from the work role may consider himself dysfunctional and feel that he cannot, or find that he does not know how to, add new positive experiences to his life. Thus, what is experienced as positive may greatly depend on cultural values, internalized social norms, and personality characteristics. Therefore, many old people who experience stress as a function of the various problem source areas may have inhibited the tendency toward life enrichment. From this point of view, counseling or working with the aged involves developing methods and approaches to reawaken the tendency toward life enrichment.

---

[3] A. J. Brok, "Existential Instrumental and Developmental Issues in Leisure Relevant to Counseling and Applied Human Development," *Society and Leisure* **3**, (1976): 61–71.

[4] E. Waters, S. Fink, and B. White, "Peer Group Counseling for Older People," paper presented at the 83rd annual convention of the American Psychological Association, Chicago, Ill., 1975.

characteristics
of the enriched person

If we are to counsel or work toward the development of any goal, it is helpful to be guided by some criteria for defining the enriched person. The enriched individual adds positive experiences by:

1. Successfully resolving developmental crises and tasks as they emerge.
2. Constructing his life (passivity is not his principal mode of relating to the world).
3. Functioning as an open system—he seeks new information and considers new ideas.
4. Continuing to make an impact on others.
5. Becoming involved in activities that he considers subjectively meaningful.
6. Developing a differentiated ego structure linked to a consistent core self.
7. Maintaining a sense of spontaneity instead of being driven by impulsive actions.
8. Keeping a sense of humor that can be shared with others.

The above criteria are meant as guidelines, not as an all-inclusive list. We shall now further explain their meaning.

Successfully resolving developmental crises and tasks as they emerge. Following Erikson's and other developmental theories, we note that the personality-shaping experiences people are confronted with keep on changing throughout the life span. Many of these experiences are, in fact, not age-related but are situation-related, and thus they may repeat themselves at various points in the life cycle. For example, according to Erikson, the older person who, upon reviewing his life, feels that it has generally been worthwhile may be successfully resolving the developmental crisis of integrity versus despair, but that same person may also be faced with the recurring crises of intimacy versus isolation because of the death of a spouse or the loss of good friends.

Constructing one's life. The construction analogy implies a sense of building upon a foundation that is continuously elaborated upon as life goes on. This is not the same as the maturational concept of "growth" that implies a natural uninfluenced development. The construction analogy implies that the person needs to feel some involvement in and responsibility for his own growth. That is, he in part constructs his life. Working with the aged often involves helping people reexperience this feeling. Presumably, the person who continues to experience life this way will feel a combined sense of growth, development, and change. In short, he will feel that he is enriching his life.

Functioning as an open system. An open system denotes the ability to acquire and be influenced by new information. An individual who functions as an open system has the opportunity to continue enriching his life with those nutriments that add to his growth and development. That is, he seeks and considers new information about himself and his relation to the world. Without this ability the person cannot change, and thus the possibility of growth and development is stopped. A closed system is a system that does not accept new information. It is as if there were a permanent barrier preventing new information from entering (see Fig. 11.1). The person who functions as a closed system may be characterized as living in another cultural period or historical era—as if he needs to maintain the world outlook that characterized life at an earlier age.

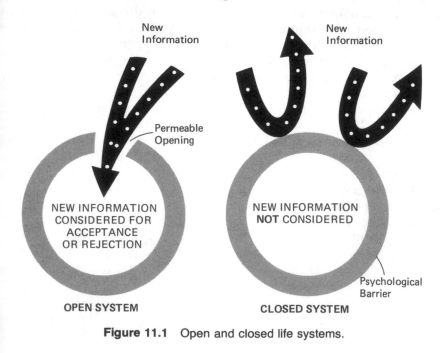

Figure 11.1 Open and closed life systems.

One example of a closed system was described by an acquaintance who told the story of his aged aunt who supported him through college. Upon his graduation she strongly tried to influence him to take a job in a "safe" civil service profession instead of going into the computer programming field, which was then a relatively new profession (this was in the early 1960's). The reason for her feelings was that she vividly recalled the depression of the 1930's and remembered how most people in business lost their jobs and that those in the civil service were relatively secure. This set of values may have been relevant in the 1930's but perhaps it was no longer so in light of the relative affluence of the 1960's (nor in the 1970's for that matter, with the increased layoffs experienced in the formerly secure civil service occupations). It seemed to him that his aunt had not allowed new information (in the area of business) to "enter in" since the depression and that she had retained a depression psychology.

Continuing to make an impact on others. This notion implies that ultimately we are social beings and that we need a sense of relationship with others in order to feel that our lives are being enriched. The quality of the relationship may be very important. Thus, a social relationship (such as playing checkers) may be pleasant, but it does not necessarily lead to a sense of enrichment. One important qualitative aspect is implied by the term *impact.* This term connotes the sense of experiencing oneself as making an impression that is clearly (as if physically) perceived in terms of the reaction of some other to one's thoughts, feelings, or actions. The term impact as used here is neutral. That is, another's reaction to what we say, do, or think may be either positive, negative, or merely acknowledged in some clear way. The crucial aspect is that what we say, do, or think is given some import, i.e., the other responds to our encounter as an open system. When this occurs we feel that we have entered into another's area of experience. Such a feeling may provide a sense of well-being. This situation, of course, should work reciprocally. Thus, the enriched person feels that he is part of the social community if his words, thoughts, or actions are given due consideration (whether they are agreed with or disagreed with). It is only when we are ignored and/or ignore others that we begin to feel isolated and alienated; such experiences can provide avenues for various forms of psychological retreat and withdrawal.[5]

---

[5]H. Guntrip, *Schizoid Phenomena, Object-Relations and the Self* (New York: International Universities Press, 1969).

Problems arise, however, when the role and the self are not linked together. Thus, the individual who overidentifies with the role of worker, as if it were not linked to a core self, but indeed *was* the core self, will have a terrible crisis when that role is lost through retirement.

Thus, the enriched person realizes that the most he can do is lend himself to a role, that he can never totally become the role (although he may better develop his self through being in the role). This notion is especially important for the aged since they are particularly subject to role loss. From this point of view, the ingredients that enrich the lives of old people consist of new ways of experiencing and differentiating their ego structure through which to express the basic core self. Expression of the core self can occur through new leisure, work, family, or community experiences.

Maintaining a sense of spontaneity.   Spontaneity should be distinguished from *impulsiveness.* Although both an impulsive and a spontaneous act are characterized by little thought, they are distinguishable in terms of how they are experienced. An impulsive activity has a "driven" quality, i.e., the person feels that the impulse must be acted upon. If it is not acted upon, there is a strong sense of frustration or discomfort.

Impulses meet certain unsatisfied needs that may be either conscious or unconscious. A spontaneous act is experienced as the product of free choice in that the individual feels free to either act or not act upon his choice. There is no sense of conflict within him; there is no blockage. If he chooses not to act, there is no strong sense of frustration. The person feels ready but does not have to do any particular thing. It seems that the tendency toward spontaneity depends on feeling comfortable and secure in one's social and psychological world. As people age, they may lose their sense of spontaneity. We suggest that it is important to maintain this sense of spontaneity and that those who work with the aged should find ways to reawaken this feeling. This might be done through leisure or other forms of group counseling.

Keeping a sense of humor that can be shared with others.   The ability to laugh at oneself and with others is perhaps a unique human ability. Humor helps relieve the seriousness of life and provides a validation that both the world and the self are to be enjoyed. By humor we do not mean cynical self-deprecating humor or the humor of denial. We mean the ability to accept the world as not only a serious place and being able to validate this feeling with peers. The two important basic abilities involved in our meaning of humor are the following:

1. The ability to appreciate or laugh at someone else's humor.
2. The ability to self-generate humor (such as telling jokes, etc.).

Most people seem to have fully developed the first ability, but the second ability, the ability to self-generate humor, is sometimes more difficult for many individuals to develop.

In sum, we suggest that humor is important because it adds to the joy of life and the feeling of well-being. Thus, working with the community aged should mean going beyond helping them deal with only serious life tasks. It may be equally as crucial to help them develop a sense of humor.

The Life Enrichment Counseling Approach

The life enrichment counseling approach is a structured counseling module.[10] The module focuses on how to help individuals recognize problems and develop approaches to the optimal use of leisure time by means of a guided discussion format that uses structured materials. The goal is to help assess and develop the creative and satisfactory use of time for individuals at different life stages, often in terms of relevant psychosocial issues, i.e., how do we help the community aged gain a sense of identity, generativity, or integrity through the use of their leisure time? The guiding philosophy of the life enrichment approach is proactive instead of purely rehabilitative in the sense that it is aimed at helping individuals enhance their developmental potential. It is also rehabilitative in the sense that it aims to restore a person's capacities to reexperience a sense of growth and reinstate feelings of worth through group interaction with peers.

---

[10]Brok, "Existential Instrumental and Developmental Issues in Leisure Relevant to Counseling and Applied Human Development."

format

Although the format is flexible, it essentially involves the following sequence of eight possible phases:

1. Introduction of the module.
2. Self-generation of leisure activities.
3. Self-evaluation of enjoyment.
4. Assessment of developmental experiences through leisure.
5. Ecological assessment of activities.
6. Qualitative descriptions.
7. Theme-oriented discussion.
8. Individual counseling and/or follow-up.

At times, phases are added or deleted for certain populations. Phases other than the introduction of the module and self-generation of leisure activities are independent and do not have to follow in any particular sequence. For illustration purposes, we shall discuss the use of this module with a target group of community aged, for example, senior citizen center participants.

Phase 1—Introduction of the Module. The rationale for introducing the module to participants can vary, depending on the setting and the purpose. As part of a senior center program, the module may be introduced as a potentially diverting activity involving the discussion and exchange of ideas about how leisure time can be used, with the group leader acting as a moderator. The module can also be introduced as a discussion of the philosophical issues of leisure from religious or other points of view. In more clinical settings the module might be used as a structured projective method for discussion of in-depth feelings about the self. The use of the module ultimately depends on the purpose of the group and the skill of the leader. It is important that all leaders be aware that they are dealing with what can rapidly become sensitive topic areas.

Phase 2—Self-generation of leisure activities. Upon introduction, participants are presented with the first form: Self-Generation of Leisure Activities (see Appendix E). Each participant is requested to make a list of the things he does in his leisure time. There are no constraining preset categories (such as checklists, etc.). The participant is encouraged to make his list as long as he desires although it is sometimes useful to have a minimal time limit, say, 10 minutes. The reason for suggesting this minimal time limit is to allow each person sufficient time to complete his list. Creativity theory has suggested that initial thought associations to a word or concept tend to be normative or stereotyped, and that with time more unusual and perhaps creative responses will emerge.[11] This is especially true for individuals whose anxiety levels are high. Thus old people who might be more subject to internal and external stresses might need more time to really get to personal interests.

Very frequently participants will ask, "What is work and what is leisure?" It is often useful to defer this question until later discussion and let the participants decide the issue for themselves. We suggest telling participants to list whatever meets their own criteria for leisure. For example, many people put down such things as "housework," which some might consider a nonleisure activity. Nevertheless, "housework" may very legitimately be subjectively experienced as leisure by certain people. This approach is in keeping with the concept of life enrichment, i.e., that people need to construct their lives and subjectively determine the meaning of their own activities.

If the participants are the community aged (such as the young–old), the form can be self-administered. If the participants are the more impaired, the directions can be read to each person and another member of the group or the group leader can write down the participant's responses.

Phase 3—Self-evaluation of enjoyment. After describing the various ways leisure time is used, participants can be asked to evaluate the degree of enjoyment they experience when involved in each separate activity. Each individual does this by circling the number that best expresses his degree of enjoyment for each activity he has recorded in his self-generated list. The numbers to be circled are printed in the *Degree of Enjoyment* part of the Self-Generation of Leisure Activities form. These numbers range from 1 through 5, where 1 stands for "little enjoyment" and 5 stands for "much enjoyment."

---

[11]M. Wallach and N. Kogan, *Modes of Thinking in Young Children* (New York: Holt, Rinehart & Winston, 1965).

This exercise can provide a general picture of how people feel about the kinds of things they subjectively list as leisure time activities. It can provide an opportunity for subsequent discussion about specific activities that are enjoyed. This discussion also allows each participant to discover similar interests and enjoyment in others, thereby providing the opportunity for validating feelings of self-esteem and self-worth.

Phase 4—Assessment of developmental experiences through leisure. After the participants have completed their lists and their enjoyment ratings, they are presented with a list of developmental task descriptors (see Activity Gains in Appendix F). These descriptors consist of eight phrases that describe developmental stages.[12] Each respondent is asked to indicate which of the phrases best expresses what he might gain from each of the activities he listed during the self-generation phase. Theoretically, the exercise should provide the developmental meaning of each person's activity repertoire. The gains are listed by number in the first form (on the right-hand side).

Provisions can be made for respondents to indicate more than one descriptor for each activity listed. This is done by asking participants to list (under the gains column in the first form) the numbers of as many descriptors they feel apply to each leisure activity. Respondents are not required to provide descriptors for activities that do not seem to meet any of their developmental needs, as described in the second form. The descriptors in the second form are illustrative phrases. It should be clear that other descriptors may be substituted, depending on the situation and population. The descriptor approach is useful for purposes of subsequent discussion rather than for assessment. The descriptors can be read to participants who find it difficult to read or write.

Phase 5—Ecological assessment of activities. This task involves the presentation of the third form, Radius of Activities (see Appendix G). Participants are asked to look over their Self-Generation of Leisure Activities form and indicate the location in which each of the listed activities is normally carried out. Participants are asked to refer to the list of eight "locales" provided in the third form and enter the appropriate number in the "place" column provided in the first form. Participant responses may

---

[12]E. H. Erikson, *Childhood and Society*, 2nd ed. (New York: W. W. Norton & Company, 1963).

indicate the extent of the exploratory activity of each individual. The participant responses can also be used for subsequent discussions about concepts of "neighborhood" and to encourage exploratory activity.

Phase 6—Qualitative descriptions. This task requires that each participant qualitatively describe, i.e., in his own words, what he experiences in (or from) the activities he engages in. The qualitative descriptions should be written or listed in the activity gains column of the first form. This phase (as do all of the other phases) leads to phase 7, the theme-oriented group discussion.

Before we turn to phase 7, we must note that the first six phases are presented as guidelines. It has been our experience that they do not have to be followed rigidly. In many cases, only some of the phases may be relevant. Indeed, each phase may be carried out as a separate unit over a period of days or weeks. The appropriateness depends on the kind of group and time allowances.

Phase 7—Theme-oriented group discussion. By theme-oriented group discussion we mean a situation in which participants are encouraged to focus on themes or issues of common concern and interest. The theme-oriented group is especially useful for the beginning worker (or counselor) because the focus should remain on a tangible topic. As previously suggested, one such topic might be the various uses for leisure time. Since it is not necessary to spend a great deal of time focusing on the analyses of emotional relations within such a group, the beginning counselor is more free to focus on the task of creating an atmosphere of mutual participation and trust through which a sense of group cohesiveness may develop. The more experienced worker will find ample material for opening up emotionally laden areas if this seems appropriate and/or the participants expect such discussion. Thus, the tangible theme group provides flexibility for different counseling or educational needs.

A theme-oriented group is less stressful for aged populations because its structure provides the opportunity to share feelings and ideas about specific topics of mutual interest. For example, by virtue of each person's involvement in the series of exercises and discussions about the uses of leisure time, a sense of "connectedness" among the participants is potentially established. In general, sharing common interests provides the touching-off point for deeper discussion.

We shall now turn to some suggestions for guiding a theme-oriented group discussion in terms of the six phases previously discussed. We suggest that it is more convenient and more facilitating to have the participants arrange themselves in small groups (six or seven) by sitting in a circle or around tables.

Uses for the Self-Generated Leisure Activities form. The material generated by the participants provides the basic discussion resource for the worker or counselor. The simplest discussion technique requires asking each participant to read out loud the items he has written. This exercise encourages participants to reveal something personal and subjectively meaningful about themselves that can be shared with others. It encourages participants to see similarities in themselves and others and it enhances a sense of "connectedness" and group cohesion. As a result, an open, theme-oriented discussion can ensue about the variety of activities that people engage in. Such a discussion can serve as an icebreaker for a newly formed group of individuals in a senior citizen or other community center. Although it does reveal material of a personal nature, it also allows people the choice of not becoming involved in any underlying emotional content if they do not want to. For example, an individual does not have to read every item on his list if he chooses not to.

The material produced by the self-generated lists can also be used to develop a more philosophical or topical discussion about the use of time. In this approach, the worker's aim is to suggest that the participants discuss "what is defined as leisure and what is not." The attempt to clarify differences between work and leisure is not always simple and can often lead the participants into a stimulating discussion about the meaning given to life activities. The discussion may also help the participants understand the subjective element in each one's personal value system. This, in turn, can encourage the appreciation of differences between oneself and others.

One suggested method for implementing the above aims is to ask participants to read their lists out loud (this should be on a voluntary basis) and then discuss whether or not they agree on what is work and what is leisure. For example, the leader might ask, "Do some of you consider what anyone else describes as leisure to be work? Why? Did anyone not include what Mr. Jones put down because you thought of it as really work? How many people put down 'cleaning house' as a leisure activity? Is it leisure for some and work for others? Why? How did each of you go about defining what was a leisure actitivty? Should we all go by the same set of definitions?"

We have also noted that some people characteristically omit or prefer not to immediately discuss certain items. For example, some individuals usually leave out sex as a leisure activity. With some humor, we have sometimes suggested that this might mean that it is considered as work! In a more serious vein, focusing on the issue of sex can lead to fruitful clinical counseling discussions about an area of human functioning that is very sensitive to many old people. Thus, it has happened that a person who was embarrassed about his needs and interest in sex at an "inappropriate age" found it both easier and less anxiety provoking to change or discuss his attitudes upon discovery that others in the group found it to be an appropriate topic that could be "talked about." Thus, both the exchange of self-generated leisure items among the participants and the discussion of what is and what is not leisure can yield a number of important social learning experiences. This, in turn, may help clarify the problem source areas of who am I? (psychological), why am I? (philosophical), and feelings about social status. When others approve of one's ideas and activities, or at least suggest that they are worthy of discussion, good feelings about the self may follow.

Uses for the Self-Evaluation of Enjoyment rating.   The simplest use for the enjoyment rating material involves a slight modification of the technique described for the use of the self-generated activity lists. This modification requires that each participant (on a voluntary basis) read out loud the activities he has rated 4 or 5. Presumably, sharing these highly enjoyed activities with others should encourage the participants to experience a sense of mutuality and cohesiveness. This approach also provides the opportunity for lively discussion about the different ratings given by members who engage in similar pastimes. As such, this exercise can provide a touching-off point for in-depth discussion about the uniqueness of one's experience in retirement, etc. Not everyone adjusts the same way, and not every activity is experienced with equal affective meaning.

Leisure ought to be joyful but, unfortunately, for many it is not. If warranted, people can be asked to compare their lists for areas that show the least enjoyment (ratings 1 and 2). This exercise can open up a discussion of such problem areas as boredom, feelings about adapting to physical limitations, etc. It can also elucidate areas of unhappiness or dissatisfaction, especially if an individual has many 1 and 2 ratings. The sensitive worker can use this material for in-depth discussion about areas of psychological apprehension and can encourage problem solving. For example, the group might discuss the following: "How and in what way can individuals do more of what they enjoy or discover new enjoyments?" Sometimes low ratings involve areas of potential guilt, such as negative feelings about doing things with certain family members. This is sometimes best handled in a psychotherapeutic context.

This exercise also lends itself to other structured approaches. Individuals can be asked to sum the number of activities they rated 4 or 5 (much enjoyment) and compare them with the number they have rated 1 or 2 (little enjoyment). This procedure can lead to a fuller discussion about how participants feel about their total leisure experiences. Do some rate everything as very enjoyable? How do they manage this? Is it all attitude? Do some have neither much enjoyment nor little enjoyment (rating of 3)? Do some have mostly little enjoyment? Such an exercise can stimulate helpful support for areas of strength and can lead to problem solving by the group for individual areas of boredom. Thus, many ways of improving or changing one's situation may emerge through discussion of the structured material.

The use of enjoyment ratings can also lead to the creation of a *human resources group.*[13] This group stresses helping each member to extend his functioning to the upper limits of his potential. In the human resources group the leader focuses on the positive potential that each member has instead of on any pathology. A group leader can use the enjoyment rating scale for such a purpose by focusing discussion on those items that each member most enjoys.

The enjoyment ratings can also be used to help people compare their ideals with the actuality of their situations. This may be done by asking participants to review their high enjoyment items (those much enjoyed) and suggesting that the participants indicate when was the last time (or how often) they had actually done or experienced each particular activity. It has been our experience that people not only put down activities that they had not done for some time (or infrequently) but they even list things that they would like to do but have never done.

The goal of the exercise is to help people better live up to their ideal self-conception and/or cope with their real self. This goal can be approached by using the following basic methods:

1. The *multiple strength perception method.*
2. The *action program method.*[14]

---

[13]D. H. Blocher, *Developmental Counseling,* 2nd ed. (New York: The Ronald Press, 1974).

[14]Ibid.

The multiple strength perception method essentially requires that one person become the center of the group's attention for a particular session. The "target" person begins by enumerating and sharing with others the strengths he sees in himself as well as the factors in his life that might inhibit him from using these strengths fully. Other members then discuss their own perceptions with him.

The action program method involves having the group encourage a particular member to develop a plan (in addition to talking about what he would like to do) to increase and facilitate the development of his strengths. According to Blocher:

> Members then report back to the group the success or failures in these action programs. When difficulties are encountered the entire group works to bring their understanding and sensitivity to bear on the problem and so help remove the blocking to further development. Action programs may begin at superficial levels such as taking art or dancing lessons and move through to quite significant undertakings such as developing greater creativity or deeper personal relationships. . . . The use of public commitment and group reinforcement are major sources of gain in this model.[15]

The usefulness of this approach is illustrated by the following: In one group a participant had listed "playing the piano" as something she enjoyed greatly. When the worker discussed the various activities, it became apparent that the last time the participant actually played a piano was some 15 years ago. This was clearly an incongruency between her actual self and her ideal self. When asked why she no longer played a piano a number of important things emerged. First, it had nothing to do with physical disability. Second, and more importantly, it had been an activity that she had given only cursory thought to and she had been timid about revealing her interest in it to anyone. Yet it was something she greatly enjoyed. This exercise permitted her dormant potential to emerge. Once it emerged, the group discussion provided the opportunity for others to express interest in her activity. In addition, the participants inquired why she had not been playing the piano recently and began to motivate her to develop an "action plan." Thus, the other members became potential resources. One member recalled that a piano was available in the lounge of the small college where this discussion took place. This led to the group's considering how and when the

---

[15]Ibid., pp. 219–220.

piano could be used by our "target person" not only to play at senior citizen events but to also teach others. Thus, the group was able to activate an interest that had been lying dormant for some years. It is for this sort of purpose that the enjoyment rating technique might be most fruitfully used.

Uses for the Activity Gains form—assessment of developmental experiences through leisure.   A discussion about what is gained through involvement in the various activities that participants list can lead to reflection about their life experiences in developmental terms. The assessment technique illustrated by the Activity Gains form provides a tangible way of approaching such developmental material. The counselor or worker can use each person's self-assessment to encourage a deeper discussion about life goals. Descriptor phrases can be used to encourage a discussion about developmental life tasks in terms of the subjective experiences of the members. Since the descriptor phrases are worded in terms of positive experiences, they lend themselves for use as part of the multiple strength perception and action program methods.

One important area of life experience that the assessment of developmental experiences through leisure technique sometimes reveals is the need for intimacy (item 6). For some, intimacy emerges as a definite strength (in that a number of activities seem to meet this need). For others, it is clearly a significant deficit. We shall focus on this issue for illustrative purposes.

Confiding intimately with someone so that one's personal problems, thoughts, and feelings can be shared is highly important for older people. Kimmel, for example, notes that having a confidant might offset the depressing experience of role loss and/or decline in social interaction that is often experienced by the aged.[16] The need for intimacy is not necessarily resolved by increased participation in general social activity programs. As we noted in our discussion about the importance of continuing to have an impact on others, two people can play many games of cards or checkers without necessarily finding out much about each other. This is not to say that social activities for the aged are bad. It is only to say that the functions of these programs are useful but limited.

In light of the above, we question why many of the programs for the elderly seem to focus on implementing the dictates of activity theory. Broadly stated, activity theory involves the idea that "if you keep busy, you stay healthy." This notion, derived from the

---

[16]D. Kimmel, *Adulthood and Aging* (New York: John Wiley & Sons, 1974).

American ethic of rugged individualism in conjuncton with the
wear and tear biological theory of aging, suggests that what old
people keep busy with may be less important than the mere activity
of keeping busy.[17] Furthermore, it seems that many old people
have internalized this notion. Bengston, for example, quotes a
73-year-old who said that his only life goal was "to keep active—I
want to wear out, not rust out."[18] If this attitude is uncritically
accepted as typical by workers and programmers for the aged, it
may lead to an overemphasis on activity and to a diminished
concern with providing relationship experiences which, in the long
run, are probably more important for uplifting morale. Lowenthal
and Haven, for example, found that old people who maintained a
stable intimate relationship evidenced less depression and more
life satisfaction (morale) than did old people who reported having
no confidant. Their findings also showed that morale remained
high for those older people who had confidants even if they had
suffered decreases in role status or level of social interaction.[19]
More recently, in a study of older people who moved into a
retirement community, it was found that social activity with friends
was the only factor in any way related to reports of life
satisfaction.[20] It seems clear that the continued experience of
having an impact on others and with others is very important to the
community aged.

Thus, we believe that the *confidant theory* (or impact theory)
and its implications should be more carefully adhered to by those
who work with the aged. Broadly stated, the confidant theory holds
that keeping busy is important, but being involved with someone in
a stable relationship (with someone with whom you can share your
activities or feelings about yourself and with someone who will
share his feelings with you) is more important. Such needs, and
how well they are met, may be elucidated by the developmental
assessment exercise.

    *Uses for the Radius of Activities form—ecological assessment of
activities.*   It has often been said in old age one's spatial world

---

[17]J. A. Kuypers and V. L. Bengston, "Social Breakdown and Competence," *Human Development* **16** (1973): 181–201.

[18]V. L. Bengston, *The Social Psychology of Aging* (New York: Bobbs-Merrill Company, 1973), p. 6.

[19]M. F. Lowenthal and C. Haven, "Interaction and Adaptation: Intimacy as a Critical Variable," *American Sociological Review* **33** (1968): 20–30.

[20]B. W. Lemon, V. L. Bengston, and J. A. Peterson, "Activity Types and Life Satisfaction in a Retirement Community," *Journal of Gerontology* **27** (1972): 511–523.

shrinks because the environment is not designed to accommodate the needs of old people. For example, an old person may have difficulty crossing wide avenues because street lights change too rapidly and stairs may prevent access to subways or commuter trains. Indeed, research studies show that old people cannot take advantage of many of the numerous facilities available to younger, more mobile members of the population[21] because the environment is not geared to them. This nonuse of facilities may lead to a spatial shrinking that may be a combined function of socially induced psychological barriers (such as depression related to retirement and caution induced by a nonchallenging environment) and biological deficits associated with aging. Discounts and passes for senior citizens are not always the answer. For example, one person would not use her senior citizen pass (for public transportation and other available discounts) because the pass symbolized "admitting that she was old." She thus stopped visiting friends in distant neighborhoods and she cut down on going out because she really could not afford to pay the regular transportation fares and other prices on her social security income. Thus, some old people may need various forms of remotivational counseling to deal with the more socially induced psychological deficits in spatial mobility.

The information derived from participants who use the third form, Radius of Activities, is useful because it provides potential role models for exploring greater parts of the environment. Through discussion with peers an older person who has confined himself to a narrow radius might be influenced by someone else in the group to broaden his activity horizon. The information about what others do can also generate motivation for trying new activities. Thus, discussion of the radius of activities can provide the opportunity for various social learning experiences and it can complement the case-centered and human resources approaches previously discussed. For the young–old, ecological assessment and discussion can serve the function of remotivational counseling. For the more physically impaired, the assessment may help engender reality confrontation and discussion of how to deal with the problems of decreased mobility without giving up one's full exploratory potential. Physical immobility does not necessarily imply psychological immobility. We recall one such discussion in a nursing home that turned into a group planning session on how to

---

[21]M. P. Lawton and L. Nahemow, "Ecology and the Aging Process," in *The Psychology of Adult Development and Aging,* eds., Eisdorfer and Lawton.

arrange for transportation (through administration) for trips to a nearby city, a topic that might not have otherwise emerged.

Transportation, however, is not always a psychological problem and its high cost is not always the barrier to exploratory behavior. Carp, for example, concluded that the extensive social isolation found in her study of the elderly in San Antonio, Texas, resulted from the unavailability as well as the high cost of transportation in that city. She found that bus service routes were not within easy access and that buses either ran infrequently or did not go directly to destinations desired by many of the aged in her sample.[22] A study by Bourg in Nashville found a similar situation. He concluded that easy access to transportation was a critical link in the ability of elderly persons to remain functional members of society.[23] Similarly, of 780 New York elderly over 65 years of age who were interviewed, it was found that most of them walked a good deal both for functional activities such as shopping as well as for leisure activities: Thus:

> When asked about what they did each time they left the house during a two-day interval, 56 percent of the trips mentioned were walking trips, particularly for local shopping. Trips that necessitated leaving the neighborhood were *infrequently* undertaken.
> Relatives . . . were likely to be visited only once a month, whereas friends, who more often lived nearby, were likely to be visited more frequently. The average person estimated that he could walk about nine blocks to the store without becoming tired.[24]

The foregoing discussion points out that anyone who works with an older population must pay particular attention to the influence of environmental factors on observed behavior. This is especially so if the aim is to help motivate an exploratory attitude. The social learning and role modeling implicit in group approaches may be an avenue to achieve such an aim. Short of changing the environment, theme-oriented group discussion approaches, such as the ecological assessment technique, can help the aged break dysfunctional attitudes resulting from

[22]F. Carp, "Public Transit and Retired People," in *Transportation and Aging: Selected Issues*, eds., E. J. Cantilli and J. L. Schnelzer (Washington, D.C.: Administration of Aging, 1971).

[23]C. Bourg, "Life Styles and Mobility Patterns of Older Persons," paper presented at the Interdisciplinary Workshop on Transportation and the Aging, Administration on Aging, Washington, D.C., May, 1970.

[24]Lawton and Nahemow, "Ecology and the Aging Process," p. 656.

environmentally and socially induced feelings of decreased competence. In this light, Bengston noted that ". . . an individual's sense of self, his ability to mediate between self and society, and his orientation to competence are related to the kinds of social labeling and valuing he experiences in aging."[25]

Given the sociological fact that the aged are labeled as dysfunctional in our society, we should not be startled to discover that many of our community aged have internalized a sense of incompetence that manifests itself in decreased exploratory potential. Recall, for example, the woman who would not use her senior citizen pass because it symbolized old age (or incompetence?) which, in turn, actually made her incompetent because she cut down on visiting. In sum, the ecological assessment technique is one method devised to break this syndrome. It does so by providing the following:

1. New reference groups.
2. New role models of ecological competence.
3. An opportunity for group planning functions in relationship to the environment.

Uses of the qualitative descriptions of leisure experiences. The simplest use of the qualitative description of experiences phase is that the worker helps develop a sense of communication and understanding among participants about each others' personal life. The worker or counselor may initiate a group session by suggesting that each participant discuss and share the kinds of things he does with his leisure time. It is not necessary to require that each participant refer to his list of self-generated activities or forms such as the enjoyment rating, etc. Here the format can be more freewheeling in order to encourage general open discussion. Although this approach is simple, it adheres to the notion of tangible themes because the topic focus can remain on leisure. The qualitative description approach may be incorporated as part of the discussion of the self-generated activities list. This can be done by suggesting that participants discuss (without referring to any of the forms) and compare what they gain from each of their listed activities.

---

[25]Bengston, *The Social Psychology of Aging,* p. 47.

Phase 8—Individual counseling and follow-up.   Although not
crucial, it is sometimes fruitful to have ongoing counseling
available in order to deal more specifically with issues raised by the
leisure discussion exercises and theme groups. We suggest that the
worker be prepared to make appropriate referrals whenever the
need for more intensive counseling arises. Such referrals should
only be suggested, of course, if the participants ask for them. We
might also note that, in general, old people as a group do not want
individual counseling even when it is readily available. In this light,
the best modality for follow-up appears to be group counseling
and/or group therapy.[26]

The Peer Group Counseling Approach

Another approach to working with the community aged has
recently been developed by Waters, Fink, and White.[27] They note
that over the years researchers have consistently observed that
older people receive a very small share of available
psychotherapeutic services. Indeed, it has been suggested that
many therapists tend to avoid working with older people because
of the anxiety these clients engender because of their inevitable
physical decline. Pomeroy suggests that therapists tend to be more
reinforced by the reassurance that comes from working with
younger patients.[28] Psychoanalysts too have noted the various
difficulties that younger therapists have with an elderly
population. Grotjahn suggests that younger therapists feel
self-conscious or apologetic when they work with clients who are
much older than themselves. He suggests that therapists who wish
to treat elderly patients must have successfully analyzed their own
attitudes toward their own parents and grandparents.[29] Another
problem can occur if the therapist becomes unduly idealizing or
patronizing with his elderly clients. This playing out of the "good"
grandchild role may inevitably leave both parties uncomfortable. It
seems that the best possible attitude for any worker to maintain is

---

[26]Waters, Fink, and White, "Peer Group Counseling for Older People."
[27]Ibid.
[28]E. Pomeroy, "Group Psychotherapy in Old Age: Chance for Creative
Intervention," *Geriatric Focus,* November, 1972.
[29]M. Grotjahn, "Analytic Psychotherapy with the Elderly," *Psychoanalytic Review* **42**
(1955): 419–427.

one of warm empathetic directness. We believe that anyone who
works with the aged should be trained to deal with the potential
problem areas discussed above.

In general, it appears that help with making satisfying
interpersonal relationships has not been made readily available to
many of the aged, even though many of them report feeling lonely,
isolated, and depressed. A group counseling approach that relies
on the use and the development of paraprofessional peer
counselors has been suggested to meet these interpersonal needs.[30]
A peer counselor is someone from one's own age group who is
trained to work therapeutically (though often in a limited capacity).
A major value of peer counseling is that older counselors often
share the same life experiences as their clients. An additional value
of this approach is that the peer counselors themselves are often
helped in significant ways through the process of being trained to
perform a helping function. There seems to be little doubt that if
older community peers are trained to a level of paraprofessional
expertise, they can be very helpful in senior center programs.
According to Waters, Fink, and White, "It is difficult for clients to
say that they are too old to learn when their group counselors range
in age from 55 to 75, and are themselves clearly launched in new
directions."[31]

the continuum center model

The peer group counseling approach originated at the
Continuum Center at Oakland University in Michigan. The
program has two main purposes: to develop peer group counselors
for the community aged and to provide a direct interpersonal
counseling service to the community aged in the Detroit area. The
principal aim of the program is to help older people deal
meaningfully with issues of loneliness and alienation through the
opportunity to share their concerns with others and to develop new
and meaningful relationships through peer interaction.

The program. The initial phase of the peer group counseling
program is structured. It offers time-limited group counseling in a
series of seven 2-hour sessions. There are two stages. Following a
preorientation meeting during which the goals of the program are

---

[30]Waters, Fink, and White, "Peer Group Counseling for Older People."
[31]Ibid., p. 10.

introduced and commitments for participation are made, a series
of structured communication skills and values clarification
exercises are presented. For example, group members are asked to
place themselves at either of two sides of the meeting room as a way
of indicating which one of two pairs of words presented by the
leader in a series of dyads—such as "Cadillac or Volkswagen,"
"loner or grouper," "bubbling brook or placid lake"—they are most
like. This forced-choice exercise derived from values clarification
is a technique presumed to motivate self-exploration and
precipitate involvement.[32]

Following these initial exercises, participants are broken up
into structured small groups in which they discuss their reactions to
the previous session. According to Waters, Fink, and White:

> [At session two] . . . participants are asked to spend five minutes in
> the small group talking about people and experiences which have
> been most significant in their lives, ending with what is most
> important to them at the present time. This encourages participants
> to talk about themselves, to focus on strengths they have developed,
> and to look at and listen to each other. Throughout this exercise,
> group (peer) leaders model reflective listening.[33]

Subsequent sessions involve similar structured activities that focus
on heightening self-esteem and improving interpersonal
competence. Participants are encouraged to go on a "trust walk,"
which theoretically involves learning how to deal with depending
on someone else. The "trust walk" method requires that one
member of a pair close his eyes while being led by another member
of the group. Another typical activity performed by the group is a
"naming" exercise that requires everyone to state each member's
name every time the group meets. This "naming" exercise has
proven to reinforce further learning, for many group members
have claimed that they were able to remember all of the names even
though they thought that they were too old to learn them. The
sessions end with a strength bombardment activity.[34] In this
exercise, each person lists his strengths on a pice of paper and other
group members add strengths they have observed in that person
during the program's progress. This technique may be considered

---

[32]S. B. Simon, L. W. Howe, and H. Kuschenbaum, *Values Clarification* (New York:
Hart Publishing Co., 1972).
[33]Waters, Fink, and White, "Peer Group Counseling for Older People," p. 6.
[34]J. McHolland, *Human Potential Seminars* (Evanston, Ill.: Kendall College, 1972).

another example of a *tangible* counseling approach to working with the community aged. Unlike the life enrichment approach, peer group counseling seems to rely on structured *exercises* instead of structured *themes*.

After having participated in the exercise series, clients are provided the opportunity for less structured personal counseling in order to follow up on any issues raised during the sessions. Waters, Fink, and White report that very few of their elderly clients seek individual counseling but that approximately one-third of them continue in small group counseling. They suggest that the generally observed reluctance of older people to seek various forms of psychological help may be more related to treatment modality (the form in which treatment is available) than to other factors. Group members are also encouraged to enroll in the paraprofessional training program. Much success is reported with this latter approach.[35]

---

[35]Waters, Fink, and White, "Peer Group Counseling for Older People."

12

teaching the community about the aged

Alternatives to Institutionalization

The vast majority of elderly live in the community. Yet they are stereotyped as senile people who are institutionalized. More often than not these stereotypes are reinforced in the media. Moreover, stories about "good" care in a facility seldom make news, but scandals are insured a place on page 1. Much of the current focus in the field of aging is on providing "alternatives to institutional care." As stated earlier, only a very small proportion of the elderly are institutionalized. Thus, for the majority of the elderly, the home and the neighborhood are the central locations in their lives and, therefore, the appropriate foci for the provision of services.

Traditionally, the elderly have been expected to bring themselves to whatever service programs are offered, but they have not always come. There are many reasons for this, for example, pride; lack of knowledge; expensive and inconvenient public transportation; bureaucratic barriers such as eligibility requirements for services; long waits at clinics and other agencies; insensitive attitudes of those who render the services; fragmentation of services; and, most important, gaps in the current service delivery system. Thus, to date, many well-intentioned, well-funded programs have been woefully underutilized.

It should be stressed again that all aging persons, although chronologically similar, are *distinct individuals* who have a multitude of varied and unusual skills, abilities, and problems. Therefore, interventions must be based on understanding this distinctiveness of the aging individual. It is apparent that there is a need for a whole spectrum of services that would allow for individual adaptations by providing a range of options. One of the primary advantages of living in the community is that the individual has access to more options than does the individual who lives within the closed system of a facility. A major goal then would be to maintain this independence by providing the aging person in the community with the necessary support services that would allow him to function optimally.

An advantage to this approach that is very seldom recognized is that the cost of maintaining the aging person in the community is generally far less than that of providing the total services of an institution. Since health care budgets are limited, more services could be dispersed among more people in the community, thus stretching health care dollars. Moreover, this approach places the focus of services in the home and neighborhood, which is precisely where the target population is.

pathology in the community

There are no precise statistics available on the incidence of mental illness in the community elderly. The reasons for this are as follows:

1. Little attention has been paid to the mental health needs of the community elderly.
2. The statistics that have been collected are from mental institutions or nursing homes and thus do not reflect the elderly population in general.
3. There is no widespread agreement on exactly what mental illness in the elderly is. For example, organic brain syndrome is said to be present in perhaps as many as one-half of the patients in nursing homes.[1] Yet, according to other estimates, there are some symptoms of organic brain syndrome in one-half of the total over-65 community population. On the surface, there seems to be a contradiction. The difficulty here is one of definition. The degrees of impairment can range from mild, occasional forgetfulness to total disorientation.

---

[1] R. W. Redich, M. Kramer, and C. A. Taube, "Epidemiology of Mental Illness and Utilization of Psychiatric Facilities Among Elder Persons," in *Mental Illness in Later Life*, eds., E. W. Busse and E. Pfeiffer (Washington, D.C.: American Psychiatric Association, 1973).

Obviously, the differences are vast between two groups of elderly, those exhibiting mild symptoms and those exhibiting severe symptoms. When the estimates are confined to those who have severe symptoms, the figures range from 4 percent to 5 percent.[2]

Nonetheless, in the past few years there has been increasing recognition that the aged experience the same mental and emotional disorders as do younger persons but probably more frequently. It is hypothesized that the increased incidence of mental and emotional problems may be related to the increasing number of stresses and losses that are experienced with increased age. However, many of the mental health difficulties of the elderly are largely treatable, as they are in younger groups. Therefore, as with any community group, the worker must be sensitive to the presence of such symptoms as depression, anxiety, and addiction. In addition, the worker must be sensitive to the myriad stresses that can precipitate emotional crises, e.g., financial problems, physical problems, bereavement, forced retirement, malnutrition, and isolation. Very often symptoms can be correlated with these external stresses and can be alleviated with appropriate interventions such as medical treatment, drugs, counseling, and psychotherapy. However, before treatment can be offered for emotional problems, there must be a physical and psychosocial assessment by qualified professionals. It must be emphasized once again that each patient is an individual. The worker should thus be alerted to the fact that aging itself is *not* a *disease* and that many of the problems of the aging are, therefore, treatable. Recognition of problems and referral to appropriate personnel are meaningful services that the worker can provide.

Needs of the Elderly

In this century we have seen a tremendous increase in life expectancy and hence a dramatic increase in the number and proportion of elderly. However, we have not seen a concomitant increase in our concern for the well-being of this segment of the population. In fact, at least 25 percent of those over 65 are now

---

[2]E. W. Busse, "Mental Disorders in Later Life—Organic Brain Syndromes," in *Mental Illness in Later Life,* eds., Busse and Pfeiffer.

living below the poverty level and many more are hovering around it, constantly struggling to make ends meet.[3]

Related to the above is the fact that we are a youth-oriented society and as such we try to deny aging as much as possible. The elderly who manage to look young and to "think young" fit in. The others remain invisible and often isolated, with both groups tending to perpetuate our society's denial of aging. Nowhere is this more apparent than in the realm of public policy. Simply put, when it comes to aging, we have none! And there has yet to be a coordinated effort to change this. Programs and services remain fragmented and inadequate. For example, social security legislation was designed to meet the post-Depression crisis of the 1930's and not to be the primary source of postretirement income that it is today. Medicare insurance was intended to make more and better health care accessible to the elderly regardless of income but, in reality, it now covers less than one-half of the annual out-of-pocket health expenditures of today's elderly and has fallen far short of its goal.[4] A multitude of similar examples can be drawn from many existing programs and services.

What, then, is needed? A sound public policy must be devised that would establish a government commitment toward making changes to improve the lot of the elderly. Needs and priorities could then be established. These needs and priorities would determine what programs and services would be established and offered. Basically, there is a need for establishing a total range of options that would insure aging people the necessary support that would enable them to maintain themselves in the community and to have, as much as possible, a continuity of life style.

Comprehensive Services

A network of comprehensive services would include simultaneous medical, social service, personal service, and environmental interventions. Available options would form a spectrum of services based on needs ranging from minimal interventions such as one-time information and referral ("I and R") services on the one

---

[3] H. B. Brotman, "Who Are the Aging?," in *Mental Illness in Later Life*, eds., Busse and Pfeiffer.

[4] R. Butler, *Why Survive?* (New York: Harper & Row, 1975).

hand to institutional placement for total care on the other. In devising this network, the following should be considered:

1. Because of the realities of increasing physical and mental frailty with increasing age and the fact that many elderly are at some point on a downhill course, there must be recognition of a *long-term need for services*. The kind of service may have to be altered as conditions change. But, no matter what the service, the goal would insure optimal functioning, however limited this might appear. The services would range from simple preventive care such as routine health screenings to the total care of the skilled nursing facility (SNF).

2. Realistic *goals* must be set. Goals in working with the elderly are often relatively *limited* and this fact must be recognized. For example, a young stroke victim may be rehabilitated to engage in contact sports, but a frail elderly person may only be rehabilitated to walk again with the help of a walker.

3. *Options* must be provided to account for individual differences. For example, housing alternatives might include single-family dwellings, apartment living, hotels, assisted apartment living (services offered in the building), communes, or other forms of congregate living, the most extreme or total being the nursing home or mental hospital. Simple activity opportunities might include the range of commercially available recreation opportunities; organizations such as church groups; organizations of retired people; public programs such as senior citizen centers; day care programs; or volunteer work and employment programs.

4. There is a need for *outreach*. A fact to be considered is that many elderly remain invisible and, therefore, isolated. These people are often the target population for services but they are rarely reached. The elderly do not generally seek out services; therefore, services must be brought to the elderly. Those who provide services must be mobile and must be able to bring the services to neighborhoods and even to the home. An example might be a mobile crisis intervention team, i.e., a team of mental health professionals which might include a psychiatrist, nurse(s), social worker(s), and other professionals and paraprofessionals who could go to the home, for example, of a distraught, emotionally troubled aging person who will not leave the house despite the efforts of caring family, friends, and neighbors.

5. There is a need for a *linkage of services*. Someone must take the initiative to coordinate the services. Currently, fragmentation is a tremendous problem. For example, an elderly client who has both physical and emotional difficulties may be treated simultaneously by several doctors who have no communication with one another. A possible consequence is that the client may be placed on contraindicated medications. Moreover, since no one physician is involved in total care and since the client may have no family and no significant others, the need for homemaking services is overlooked in the shuffle. As a result, the client may feel psychologically fragmented and thus further stress may be added. In this case, a social worker, nurse, or paraprofessional staff person at a community agency may serve as a liaison. Thus, expensive duplication of services may be avoided. This same person may also be a provider of advocacy services for the elderly client who is unable to fend for himself.

The Elderly Person
as an Advocate for Himself

Most elderly people would be their own advocates if they were given the opportunity. The complexities of the current services system, their limited education and the limited mobility of many of our elderly make them being advocates extremely difficult. This may be compounded by the fact that so many of today's aging persons were raised in an era in which activism was frowned upon as being "rabble rousing," and they passively accept their lot. (This is in contradistinction to a group of dynamic activists that champions the rights of the elderly and is known as the "Gray Panthers.") In addition, there is a tendency for many professionals as well as laymen to treat the elderly as nonpeople or at best to infantilize them, i.e., to treat them as though they were children (note the common stereotype of the old person regressing to "second childhood"). Thus, instead of listening to the client and acceding to his wishes, decisions and services are inflicted upon him. Consequently, many elderly are forced into being dependent. The more the dependency is encouraged, the more dependent they become, thus creating a vicious cycle.

To break this cycle, a massive program of education for aging is indicated. This program should include a generalized education that would start with young children and would present aging as a developmental stage not very different from other stages in the life cycle. Special efforts should be made to reach middle-aged persons and to encourage them to actively attempt to improve the lot of their parents while simultaneously assuring a better future for themselves. Again, the professionals and paraprofessionals who are currently working with the aged could and should serve as change agents in this process. Most of all, the elderly themselves should be included in this process because they could help dispel some of the negative stereotypes and myths about aging by providing direct evidence of the positive attributes of aging that can be maximized through *direct interaction* between aging persons and the community at large. To educate for *aging* is to educate for *life.*

appendix
evaluation
forms

A

geriatric rating scale

Instructions

Rate each patient by circling either a zero, one, or two after each item. The *higher* the score the *less* intact is the patient's functioning. Thus, a high score (many ratings of 2) would indicate that a patient is functioning poorly and could be assigned to a rehabilitative program such as sensory training. Where the patient's scores fall in the medium range (many ratings of *1*) he might be assigned to a program such as reality orientation. A total score which includes many zeros might indicate an approach such as remotivation or activity therapy.

Patient's Name _____

Rater's Name _____

Date _____

Circle *only* the number which applies

1. When eating, the patient requires:
   No assistance (feeds himself)   0
   A little assistance (needs encouragement)   1
   Considerable assistance (spoon feeding, etc.)   2

2. The patient is incontinent:
   Never   0
   Sometimes (once or twice per week)   1
   Often (three times per week or more)   2

3. When bathing or dressing, the patient needs:
   No assistance   0
   Some assistance   1
   Maximum assistance   2

4. The patient will fall from his bed or chair
   unless protected by side rails:
   Never   0
   Sometimes   1
   Often   2

5. With regard to walking, the patient:
   Has no difficulty   0
   Needs assistance in walking   1
   Does not walk   2

6. The patient's vision, with or without glasses, is:
   Apparently normal   0
   Somewhat impaired   1
   Extremely poor   2

7. The patient's hearing is:
   Apparently normal   0
   Somewhat impaired   1
   Extremely poor   2

8. With regard to sleep, the patient:
   Sleeps most of the night   0
   Is sometimes awake   1
   Is often awake   2

9. During the day, the patient sleeps:
   Sometimes   0
   Often   1
   Most of the day   2

10. With regard to restless behavior at night, the
    patient is:
    Seldom restless   0
    Sometimes restless   1
    Often restless   2

11. The patient's behavior is worse at night than
    in the daytime:
    Never   0
    Sometimes   1
    Often   2

12. When not helped by other people, the patient's
    appearance is:
    Almost never sloppy   0
    Sometimes sloppy   1
    Almost always sloppy   2

	Circle *only* the number which applies

13. The patient masturbates or exposes himself
publicly:
Never   0
Sometimes   1
Often   2

14. The patient is confused (unable to find his way
around the ward, loses his possessions, etc.)
Almost never   0
Sometimes   1
Often   2

15. The patient knows the names of:
More than one member of the staff   0
Only one member of the staff   1
None of the staff   2

16. The patient communicates in any manner (by
speaking, writing, or gesturing) well enough to
make himself easily understood:
Almost always   0
Sometimes   1
Almost never   2

17. The patient reacts to his own name:
Almost always   0
Sometimes   1
Almost never   2

18. The patient plays games, has hobbies, etc.:
Often   0
Sometimes   1
Almost never   2

19. The patient reads books or magazines on the
ward:
Often   0
Sometimes   1
Almost never   2

20. The patient will begin conversations with others:
Often   0
Sometimes   1
Almost never   2

	Circle *only* the number which applies		

21. The patient is willing to do things asked of him:
    Often — 0
    Sometimes — 1
    Never — 2

22. The patient helps with chores on the ward:
    Often — 0
    Sometimes — 1
    Never — 2

23. Without being asked, the patient physically helps other patients:
    Often — 0
    Sometimes — 1
    Almost never — 2

24. With regard to friends on the ward, the patient:
    Has several friends — 0
    Has just one friend — 1
    Has no friends — 2

25. The patient talks with other people on the ward:
    Often — 0
    Sometimes — 1
    Almost never — 2

26. The patient has a regular work assignment:
    Away from the ward — 0
    On the ward — 1
    No regular assignment — 2

27. The patient is destructive of materials around him (breaks furniture, tears up magazines, etc.)
    Never — 0
    Sometimes — 1
    Often — 2

28. The patient disturbs other patients or staff by shouting or yelling:
    Never — 0
    Sometimes — 1
    Often — 2

	Circle *only* the number which applies

29. The patient steals from other patients or staff members:
    - Never — 0
    - Sometimes — 1
    - Often — 2

30. The patient *verbally* threatens to harm other patients or staff:
    - Never — 0
    - Sometimes — 1
    - Often — 2

31. The patient *physically* tries to harm other patients or staff:
    - Never — 0
    - Sometimes — 1
    - Often — 2

Total score (   )

sensory training evaluation

The following is a modified outline of the sensory training evaluation form. It was compiled with an interdisciplinary team at David Minkin Rehabilitation Institute, Brooklyn, N.Y.

Instructions

At the end of *each* session, please rate the patient on each of the areas listed. The highest number (2) indicates the best level of response and the lowest (0) the poorest level of response.

Patient's Name _____ Age _____ Sex _____

Leader's Name _____ Ward _____

Job Title _____ Date _____ Session No. _____

Does the patient speak English? well _____ poorly _____ not at all _____

	(2) Usually	(1) Sometimes	(0) Never
1. Identification of body parts (can identify by touching or verbalizing)	_____	_____	_____

	(2) Usually	(1) Sometimes	(0) Never
2. Recognition of different odors (recognizes by saying: "this is sweet, bitter," etc.)	_____	_____	_____
3. Awareness of different textures (can identify a piece of rough cloth, a piece of velvet, etc.)	_____	_____	_____
4. Auditory acuteness (attentive when others are talking)	_____	_____	_____
5. Visual attentiveness (looks at leader or other members when appropriate)	_____	_____	_____
6. General interest in others (appears interested in leader or others around him)	_____	_____	_____
7. General interest in environment (notices things around him)	_____	_____	_____
8. General enjoyment (seems to enjoy being with others)	_____	_____	_____
9. General participation (shows attempts to participate in group)	_____	_____	_____
10. General positive adaptation (e.g., is not disruptive in group)	_____	_____	_____

Total score* (   )

*To get the total score, give a weight of (2) to a rating of "usually", and a weight of (1) to "sometimes" and add all the scores.

The leader of the group should keep track of changes in these scores over time as a way of denoting progress or decline (see below). In addition, test scores may indicate early deterioration and a need for additional supportive measures.

Check Statement that Applies

Since the last report, has patient shown any

        a) improvement in meetings?   Yes _____   No _____
        b) improvement on the unit?   Yes _____   No _____

Final Report for Series

Initial score (first session) _____Date _____
Final score (sixth session) _____Date _____

Check off the following:

_____ Promote to higher-level group (e.g. Reality Orientation)
_____ Continue in the same group for another 6-session series
_____ Transfer to another group
_____ Inactive (to be reassigned)

Note: At final session of series, place this form on patient's chart.

C

reality orientation evaluation

The following is a modified outline of the Reality Orientation Evaluation Form. It was compiled with an inter-disciplinary team at David Minkin Rehabilitation Institute, Brooklyn, N.Y.

Instructions

At the end of *each* session, please rate the patient in every area listed. The highest number (2) indicates the best level of response and the lowest (0) the poorest level of response.

Patient's Name _____ Age _____ Sex _____

Leader's Name _____ Ward _____

Job Title _____ Date _____ Session No. _____

Does the patient speak English? Well _____ poorly _____ not at all _____

	(2) Usually	(1) Sometimes	(0) Never
1. Orientation to person (knows who he is)	_____	_____	_____
2. Orientation to place (knows where he is)	_____	_____	_____

	(2) Usually	(1) Sometimes	(0) Never
3. Orientation to time/date/day (knows the time of day, names the day, etc.)	_____	_____	_____
4. Verbal communication (responds to or initiates verbal exchange with others)	_____	_____	_____
5. Social behavior (recognizes group leader, smiles in recognition, extends hand, nods, etc.)	_____	_____	_____
6. General interest in others (appears interested in leader or others around him)	_____	_____	_____
7. General interest in environment (notices things around him)	_____	_____	_____
8. General enjoyment (seems to enjoy being with others)	_____	_____	_____
9. General positive adaptation (e.g., is not disruptive in the group)	_____	_____	_____
10. General participation (shows attempts to participate in group)	_____	_____	_____

Total score* (   )

*To get the total score, give a weight of (2) to a rating of "usually" and a weight of (1) to "sometimes" and add all the scores.

Changes in scores over time denote progress or decline. In addition, early deterioration may be noted and additional intervention measures introduced.

Check Statement that Applies

Since the last report, has patient shown any,

    a) improvement in meetings?   Yes _____   No _____
    b) improvement on the unit?   Yes _____   No _____

Final Report for Series

Initial score (first session) _____Date _____
Final score (sixth session) _____Date _____

Check off the following:

_____ Promote to higher-level group (e.g., remotivation)
_____ Continue in the same group for another 6-session series
_____ Transfer to another group
_____ Inactive (to be reassigned)

Note: At final session of series, place this form on patient's chart.

remotivation evaluation

The following is a modified outline of the Remotivation Evaluation Form. It was compiled with staff members of an inter-disciplinary team at David Minkin Rehabilitation Institute, Brooklyn, New York.

Instructions

At the end of *each* session, please rate the patient in every area listed. The highest number (2) indicates the best level of response and the lowest (0) the poorest level of response. Do this *as soon after* each session as possible.

Patient's Name _____ Age _____ Sex _____

Session No. _____ Ward No. _____ Date _____

Remotivator _____ Topic _____

Job Title _____

	(2) Usually	(1) Sometimes	(0) Never
1. Interest	_____	_____	_____
2. Awareness	_____	_____	_____
3. Participation	_____	_____	_____

	(2) Usually	(1) Sometimes	(0) Never
4. Comprehension	_____	_____	_____
5. General enjoyment	_____	_____	_____
		Total score* ( )	

*To get the total score, give a weight of (2) to a rating of "usually" and a weight of (1) to "sometimes" and add all the scores.

Check Statement that Applies

Since the last report, has patient shown any,

    a) improvement in meetings?   Yes _____   No _____
    b) improvement on the unit?   Yes _____   No _____

Final Report for Series

Initial score _____Date _____
Final score (sixth session) _____Date _____

self-generation of leisure activities

Age _____

Sex _____

Instructions

List below the kind of things which you do in your leisure time. Put down anything that comes to your mind. The order in which you write these activities is not important. After you have listed everything that you can think of, rate each activity according to a scale of enjoyment, from *1* to *5*, where *1* is the low end of the scale and *5* is the high end of the scale. Circle the number which expresses your degree of enjoyment.

Leisure Activities	Place	Degree of Enjoyment Little Much					Gains
A		1	2	3	4	5	
B		1	2	3	4	5	
C		1	2	3	4	5	
D		1	2	3	4	5	
E		1	2	3	4	5	
F		1	2	3	4	5	

Leisure Activities	Place	Degree of Enjoyment Little			Much		Gains
G		1	2	3	4	5	
H		1	2	3	4	5	
I		1	2	3	4	5	
J		1	2	3	4	5	
K		1	2	3	4	5	
L		1	2	3	4	5	
M		1	2	3	4	5	
N		1	2	3	4	5	
O		1	2	3	4	5	
P		1	2	3	4	5	
Q		1	2	3	4	5	
R		1	2	3	4	5	
S		1	2	3	4	5	
T		1	2	3	4	5	

F

activity
gains

1. This activity gives me the feeling that other people support me in my interests. My confidence in others is confirmed.

2. This activity gives me freedom to be separate and a sense of standing on my own two feet. This activity reinforces the belief of being able to take care of myself.

3. This activity gives me a chance to explore and be creative. I enjoy this activity because there are no set rules. I decide what the activity consists of and how I will do it.

4. This activity gives me a sense of accomplishment and helps me gain a sense of achievement.

5. This activity helps me to learn more about myself and helps me find out who I am. It gives me a chance to try different ways to do things and to discover new things about myself.

6. This activity allows another person to find out more about me, and encourages me to find out more about another person in depth. It involves sharing meaningful feelings with another. Through this activity I get close to another person, and expose my personal side.

7. This activity allows me to feel that I am contributing something worthwhile to others or to society. This activity helps me feel that I am giving something, that I am helping others, or that I am making my mark on another person's life, on an organization, or community.

8. Through this activity I can appreciate the differences among people and accept myself and others with our differences. This activity helps me feel satisfied with the way in which I have led my life.

Check off the following:

_____ Promote to higher-level group (e.g., discussion)
_____ Continue in the same group for another 6-session series
_____ Transfer to another group
_____ Inactive (to be reassigned)

Note: At final session of series, place this form on patient's chart.

ecology format — radius of activities

Instructions

On the first page, you have provided me with a number of activities which you do in your free time. Please note next to the activity the locale (place) you would normally do this activity. Choose from the list of 8 places below. You may use a place as often as you like or not at all.

1. Home
2. On my block
3. Within 5-block area of home
4. Neighborhood
5. Other neighborhood in town or city
6. State
7. Outside the state
8. Outside the United States

index

R

RNA, 19
Radius of activities form, 190–192
Ramm, D., 8
Reaction time, 8
Reality, bridges to, 117
Reality orientation, 63, 65, 206
  activities for, 99
  association, 99–100
  environmental destruction of, 67 (*see also* Institutionalization)
  family involvement in, 100–101
  institutional routine and, 103–105
  introducing program, 105
  leader's role in, 96–97
  leadership techniques in, 101–103
  materials for, 93–95
  movement to higher levels of, 106–107
  progress charting, 107–108
  reinforcement in, 95–96
  sessions, 92–93
  twenty-four-hour program, 98–99
Reality orientation board, 94–95
Recordkeeping, 89
  group therapy sessions, 166–167
  for reality orientation, 107, 108
  patients' recreational activities, 157
  remotivation sessions, 139–140 (*see also* Forms)
Recreation, 206
  activities, 150–154
  availability of, 155
  chance for independence through, 149
  goals of, 154–155
  schedule, 156
Refreshments, role of, 76, 95–96
Regression, 64, 146, 147
Rehabilitation:
  consistency, 142
  intervention for, 64 (diagram)
  personnel involved, 63
  step-ladder approach to, 64–65
  team approach to, 142–143
  techniques for:
    characteristics of, 63
    reality orientation, 91–112
    remotivation, 113–140
    sensory training, 63–84
Reinforcement, 82, 102
  compliments as, 136
  refreshments as, 76, 95

Reinforcement (*cont.*)
  verbal, 137
Reminiscence, 29, 117
Remotivation, 63, 65, 68, 206
  goals, therapeutic, 113–114
  as interaction stimulus, 136, 137
  materials for, 116
  recorded session of, 118–125
  sessions of, 114–115, 117–118
  structuring of, 117–118
  topics suitable for group, 135
Remotivation technician, 115–116
Repetition:
  nonverbal, 85
  as rehabilitation technique, 88, 101, 111
    (*see also* Rehabilitation techniques)
Response, securing patient, 138
Retirement, 15, 34, 38 (*see also* Aging, social; Income)
Risk taking, 41–44 (*see also* Leisure)
Richman, Leona, 69
Rivlin, L. G., 44, 46
Rosenbaum, M., 157
Role, social, 35–36, 178
Routine, institutional, 103–105
Rusting, fear of, 12

S

Sack, A., 59
Safety, physical, 47 (*see also* Certainty; Risk taking)
Sander, M., 93
Schaie, K. W., 34, 44
Schedules, as reality vehicles, 104
Scott, T. H., 62
Self:
  psychic organization of, 24
  relation to role, 178–179 (*see also* Retirement)
Self-conception, methods for achieving, 187–188
Self-esteem, 59, 60, 196
Senescence, cumulative errors leading to, 19
  (*see also* Aging, physiological)
Senile dementia, 62
Senility, spiral of, 59
Sensory training, 63, 66, 67, 206
  definition of, 65
  exercises for, 78–84

Y

Young old, 171 (*see also* Life span)
Youth, cultural emphasis on, 4 (*see also* Aging, attitudes toward)

Z

Zilboorg, G. A., 11
Zusman, J., 57